Professional Ethics
for
Audiologists
and
Speech-Language
Pathologists

AF411687

Professional Ethics for Audiologists and Speech-Language Pathologists

David M. Resnick, Ph.D.
Director, Hearing and Speech Center
Washington Hospital Center
Washington, DC

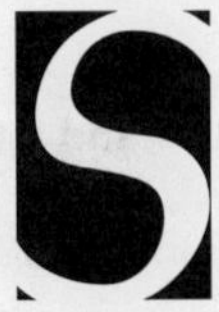

Singular Publishing Group, Inc.,
San Diego, California

Singular Publishing Group, Inc.
4284 41st Street
San Diego, California 92105-1197

© 1993 by Singular Publishing Group, Inc.

Typeset in 10/12 Palatino by So Cal Graphics
Printed in the United States of America by McNaughton & Gunn

All rights, including that of translation, reserved. No part of this publication may be reproduced, stored in a retrieval system or transmitted in any form or by any means, electronic, mechanical, recording, or otherwise, without the prior written permission of the publisher.

Library of Congress Cataloging-in-Publication Data

Resnick, David M.
    Professional ethics for audiologists and speech-language pathologists / by David M. Resnick.
        p.   cm.
    Includes bibliographical references and index.
    ISBN 1-56593-087-8
    1. Speech therapists—Professional ethics. 2. Audiologists—Professional ethics.   I. Title.
RC428.5.R48   1993
174'.2—dc20   92-34723
                                                                                      CIP

Contents

Foreword

Truth has no special time of its own. Its hour is now—always
(Albert Schweitzer—*Out of my Life and Thought*, 1949)

This is a book about professionalism, about the ethical concepts that separate professionalism from commercial pursuits. Increasingly, audiologists and speech-language pathologists find themselves in situations where conscience seems to be challenged. Is it right to accept gifts from hearing-aid manufacturers? Is it right to accept payment of travel expenses to participate in seminars and other educational activities? Is it right to engage in purchasing schemes where the program rewards large purchases with credit toward future purchases? Is it right to accept financial support for a workshop from an agency that sells goods or services involved in the workshop? What about hospitality suites at conventions? Or letting a manufacturer's representative take you to lunch?

In this book, you will not find simple and straightforward answers to these kinds of difficult questions for the very good reason that there are no simple and straightforward answers. What you will find, however, is the key to the puzzle. In a seductive and compelling manner Resnick leads us through a series of actual examples, to the inevitable conclusion that answers to difficult ethical questions cannot be imposed on us by any outside authority. They must come from within ourselves. Codes of ethical conduct cannot tell us what to do. They can only help us to realize, within ourselves, what is the right thing to do.

When you have absorbed this message, and truly understood it, you will have grasped the essence of professionalism. Good reading!

James Jerger

Acknowledgment

This is to acknowledge, that is, admit to several things over and above the help given by a number of precious people I cherish. Among these folks I even include a troublemaker or two who have repeatedly asked why in the world I was putting myself in the breach by authoring a book on ethics.

High on the list and separate from everyone else, of course, fall the editors who are true genetic throwbacks to Job. Patience is indeed a virtue, and virtue, it is said, is the beginning of ethics. Perhaps we all have experienced a common bond after all.

If each of the several people who assisted me through this endeavor is looking for a name on this page—don't. No one will be named here because I fear having to cope with the thought that someone is omitted from the list. Besides, you all know who you are, and so do I. Should anyone ask, you can tell them what you did, if you wish. Be assured that I will tell them who you are if I am asked, too. But, I will probe their intentions first. Trust me on that; I have no self-interest here, I hold *your* welfare paramount.

The chances are that the writer of a book on professional ethics focusing on a single profession or two will not make a lot of new friends. It is equally probable that some old friends will be lost as well. I acknowledge these possibilities as distinctly a conflict of interest both in appearance and in fact and directly related to the writing of this book. The choice was difficult, but it was made in your best interest—perhaps.

I have learned, after trudging through the morass of matters ethical, that ethics is a many-faceted jewel to be appreciated from a variety of angles and under an array of different illuminations. I acknowledge having succumbed to the sparkle of that jewel during the undertaking of this book. I admit to looking, but never really seeing it under any light before. Continuing education can be fun at any age!

I recognize, nonetheless, that no one who finishes reading this book will experience the same level of relief that I did when the writing of it was over—although they might. I also freely admit to a new respect for other people who write books and certainly for those who publish them.

A comment must be made about the nine or ten cartoons dispersed throughout the pages as a means devised by the editors of "breaking up the seemingly endless print" (ahem!). I would like to acknowledge that they were drawn by my good friend Gary Larson, creator of *The Far Side*. But he isn't and they weren't; so I can't. The ethical approach is to tell you I did them myself and take full blame if you should laugh—or not.

I would like at this point to acknowledge, too, the support of my family, but I'm not certain they remember I was even writing a book. After initially agreeing to my involvement in authoring a publication of book proportion my wife never said another word about it. Perhaps that was her way of not interfering. It worked. I'm done.

My daughters thought that my time in the den with the computer was spent playing Scrabble. I shall be gentle with them and merely place a copy of this book on the coffee table in my house. Perhaps one of them will pick it up one day, riffle the pages and exclaim, "Look, Mom. Dad wrote a book! And he *drew* in it, too!" Perhaps not.

Finally, I recognize that those who believed I could string enough words together to write a publishable book on ethics for the audiology and speech-language professions might be disappointed with what they see in the pages that follow. I also realize the opposite may very well be true instead, and freely acknowledge that I sincerely hope it is.

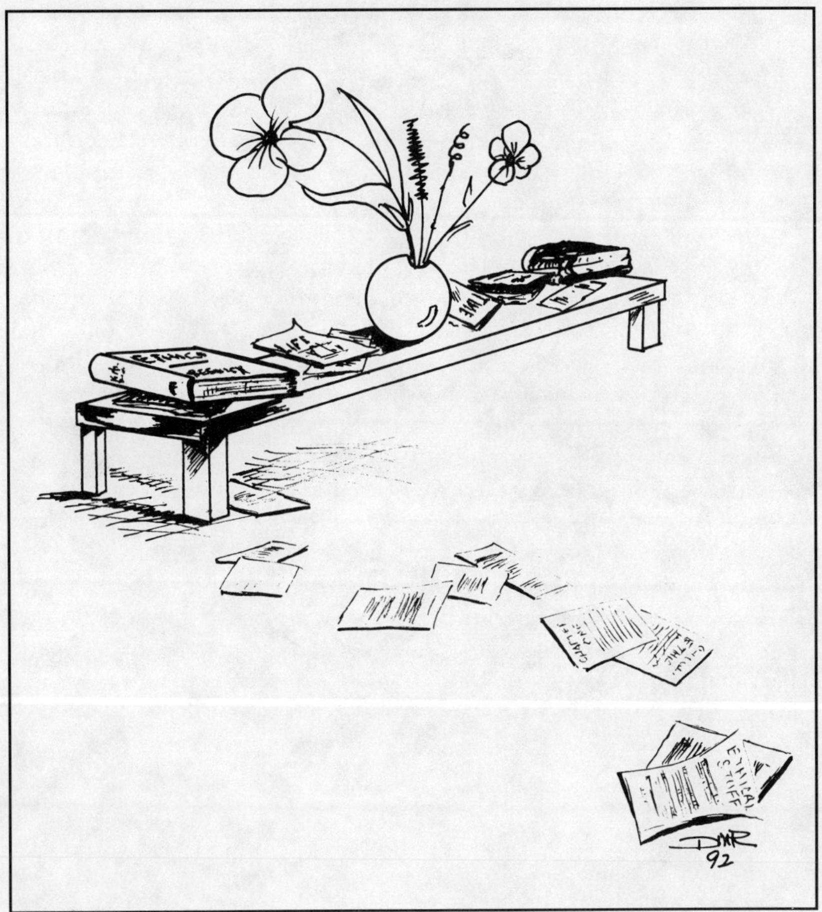

Preface

Why a book on professional ethics? One reason is that there is a strong notion that practice of the traditional professions, such as medicine, law, nursing, education, psychology, dentistry, ministry, and the like, is undergoing change because of marketplace pressure and the temptations and great advancements of the 21st century. To many professional organizations the erosion of long-entrenched ethical standards looms as a real and frightening threat. Some, including the prestigious American Medical Association, for example, have publicly indicated concern of the need for practitioners to be aware of the temptations of business and the requirement to balance the demands of commercial enterprise and professional practice in a way that preserves professional image.

Now most hospitals throughout the country have bioethics committees charged with the monumental responsibility of judging who should receive expensive methods of treatment, organ transplants, and the potential benefits of experimental procedures; who should live and the quality of that saved life; and who, for that matter, should even participate in the decision. Bioethics is a buzz word, and bioethical judgments are important to the reputation of hospitals and to the individuals who constitute the committees, as well as to society in total. The moral, philosophical, and ethical problems faced by bioethics committees are among the most difficult questions society asks of its members.

This book, however, is not about the bioethics of who should live and who should be allowed to die, or the ethics of human understanding that surrounds those God-like decisions so necessary in the midst of great scientific and technologic progress. It is not about the agonizing deliberations required of medical, religious, bioethical, and lay people over society's tough questions. The matter of bioethics is a special discipline. It requires a special touch, unique training, compassion, and indoctrination. Bioethics is outside the scope of this book, and beyond the training, skills, and perhaps even the understanding of its author.

The book **is** about ethics in a more general sense. It addresses the need for professionals to understand ethics and its imprint on the conduct of a practitioner and the image of a profession. That, then, is yet another reason for a book about ethics. This book will meet the need for audiologists and speech-language pathologists, among others, to know something about professional ethics from a practical standpoint, too. From theory to practicality the reader might even have a little fun along the way.

In a sense ethical theory involves many aspects of morality that embody a history and a code of learnable rules. Early in life people learn moral rules along with other important social rules. Later in life, however, it becomes difficult to distinguish between the moral rule and the ethical principle.

Morality is studied through a variety of methods. Not all fall into the realm of ethical theory—but some do. Two ethical theories describe and analyze without taking moral positions and are referred to as "nonnormative" approaches to ethical theory. Two others clearly do involve moral positions and are described as "normative" approaches. The categories do not define differences, however, and the four approaches are often undertaken jointly in examining the ethics of a particular issue. The distinctions are important to this book, however, because of the changes appearing in health care provisions—changes that will surely affect the professions and their ethical basis.

First among the two nonnormative fields of inquiry into morality is *descriptive ethics*, which is the factual description of moral belief. Anthropologists, sociologists, and historians employ this method when they study how moral attitudes, codes, and beliefs vary from person to person or from one society to another. A common example is the sociological study of biomedical research involving human subjects and the standards of informed consent used in conducting that research.

A second nonnormative field, *metaethics*, involves the analysis of the central terms in ethics, such as "right," "obligation," "good," "responsibility," and "virtue." The structure or logic of moral reasoning is examined in metaethics.

General normative ethics attempts to defend basic virtues and principles that govern moral life. It is an ethical theory providing a system of reasons for adopting certain moral principles. The principles found in general normative ethics are applied to moral problems such as racial and sexual discrimination, widespread hunger, abortion, or, again, research involving human subjects.

When the principles are applied in this way, *applied ethics* is being involved. Philosophical treatments of medical ethics, engineering ethics, journalistic ethics, the ethics of the law, and professional ethics all involve an application of general ethical principles to moral problems that arise in these professions.

The same general ethical principles apply to problems across professional fields and in areas beyond. One might, for example, appeal to principles of justice to resolve issues of taxation, criminal punishment, or health care distribution. Principles of truthfulness might apply to balanced reporting in journalistic ethics, misleading advertising in business ethics, or the disclosure of information to or about a patient in medical ethics, appearances of impropriety in the ethics of all professions. Applied ethics is the primary philosophy followed in this book. Its application is well suited to the context of professional ethics.

Another rationale for a book on professional ethics is that little about professional ethics is taught in the graduate programs of audiology or speech-language pathology. The ethical practice of the professions of audiology and speech-language pathology is taken for granted. Because much of the origin of professional ethics comes from the field of medicine, the ethics of that learned profession serves, to a wide extent, as a model. The view seems to be that professional ethics come naturally to professional people. Ethics just happens, some believe. There is, after all, strong evidence in history that good and lasting leaders were ethical people, or maybe it is the other way around.

There is also the belief that most ethics start with growing into and through childhood. The Golden Rule, taught early, is incontestable. It is certainly a good thing to live by: "Do unto others as you would have them do unto you."

But as children, most of us needed also to be taught that we shouldn't take what doesn't belong to us, we shouldn't lie, and we should never cheat. Some of us were taught that we shouldn't hit our sister, either. Some of us did anyway—but never really hard.

Of course, if the Golden Rule concept was not quite enough to assure good and ethical behavior, there were the Commandments— ten of them, with a bit more sting. But some of us hit our sister despite even these more powerful guideposts.

Perhaps those small childhood deviations were an oversimplified beginning of the erosions noticed in society today. Perhaps not. But there is little doubt that ethical standards have decayed in society. It is almost accepted that one may cheat a little bit, as long as one is not caught. Today the consumer wonders what the difference is between the salesman who pressures a customer into buying two items when one is sufficient and the physician who owns the X-ray machine and orders X-rays for every patient.

In part, at least, the difference once was that professions are built on trust, as well as expertise, and it was always believed that professionals were immune to compromise of that trust, no matter what. But everyday professions, too, are subject to the virus attacking ethical standards.

Intentional transgressions within the array of professions make headlines and are regularly highlighted on the nightly news. Ethical behavior is at once the most valuable quality of a profession, and at the same time it is the most vulnerable to contamination.

As the temptation increases for professions to become more like businesses because of the many societal pressures, there is the greater potential for professionals to act like business people and to be more keen on self-interest than on the welfare of the people they serve. Protection from the contamination of the virus is not absolute, and the choices open to professions interested in the preservation of trust are few. To make matters more difficult there is need for balance between the two interests—a balance that is difficult to sustain no matter how necessary it becomes.

The measure of a civilization is the care it takes of its children, elderly, poor, and sick. According to some, the United States as a nation does not measure very well in this regard. To others the United States meets a high standard. How **does** one resolve the dilemma in ethics of providing health care, for example, to some 31 million Americans who lack health insurance coverage versus leaving our children with trillions of dollars of national debt? Should such decisions be based on "logic," or instead on what is "right" or "good," or what is "ethical," or what is good business; and what is the best way to ensure that the decision is couched in something other than self-interest?

Today there are professions interested in grappling with questions such as these. Many professions in the 21st century are eager to examine what their role in the larger society needs to be. The   professional leadership sees a responsibility beyond the traditional requirements of balancing a budget, providing services to its membership, and lobbying for preservation of government support. Professions today are primarily interested in serving, not in being self-serving. That is an important distinction—it is one that sets a profession aside from all other work endeavors.

Another distinction is a code of ethics. Ethics, in general, is the practice of human conduct according to certain specified principles. The Code of Ethics of the American Speech-Language-Hearing Association, for example, states in part, that members of the Association "hold paramount the welfare of persons served professionally." The Code of Ethics of the American Academy of Audiology, as another example, indicates among other things, that its members "shall not limit the delivery of professional services on any basis that is unjustifiable, or irrelevant to the need for the potential benefit from such services." The medical ethic, in essence, tells physicians *primum non nocere*, above all do no harm. By contrast the code of ethics of the International Hearing Society, a trade organization, states in part that members pledge to "provide the best possible service to the hearing impaired," in essence a platitude not easily measurable.

As ethics is not a topic often included in many graduate school curricula, it is not unusual that many practitioners are familiar with only a few specifics about professional ethics. This needs to be changed, and that is yet another reason for a book about professional ethics. More and more, professions are being asked to document interest in, knowledge of, and actions concerning the ethical practice of the disciplines. Granting agencies are asking for it; the courts are asking for it; the government, boards of education, but, most importantly, the consumer is demanding that professionals live up to the ethics of their professions. It is time for a renewal of trust.

Ethics on an individual level means behaving in ways that demonstrate genuine concern for the well-being of people without the motivation of self-interest. At an organizational level that perspective leads to plans and deeds that empower others—association members, the consumers of their services, and the larger community in which they exist. It is in everyone's best interest to understand the ethics of professionalism, so. . . .

Why *not* a book on professional ethics?

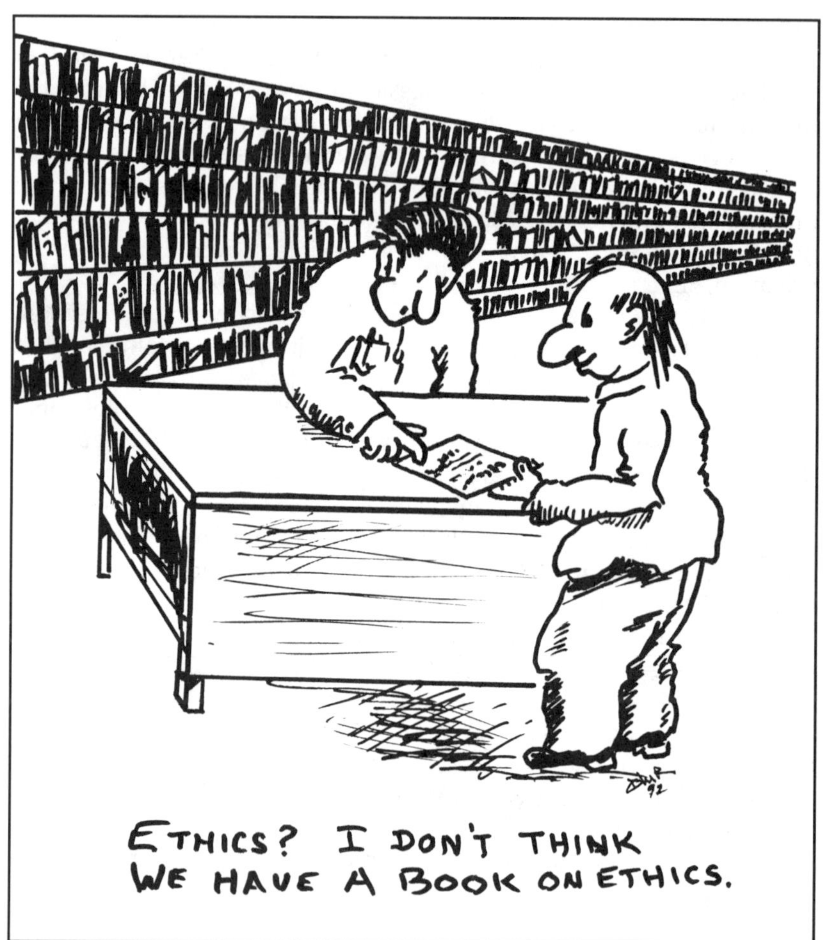

ETHICS? I DON'T THINK
WE HAVE A BOOK ON ETHICS.

1

An Introduction to Ethics

Always do what is right. That will satisfy most people and astonish the rest. (Mark Twain)

Ethics is a peculiar word. It means different things to different people, and to a few people it means very little. It refers to a lot of things most often, but sometimes it refers to only one. To make matters even more confounding the dictionary *(Webster's New World, 1984)* lists "ethics" as a plural noun to be used with a singular verb—much of the time. This would be the case in a statement such as, "The professional ethics of the American Academy of Audiology *is* under investigation," hypothetically speaking, for example. However, "Good work ethics *are* an advantage to workers in the stenographers pool," is also considered correct grammatical structure. In the one instance, conduct of members of a professional society is being treated as unified and belonging to a single code. In the other, behaviors are referred to as multiple and varied across all people in the pool, but quite good in each worker.

The distinction is a minor one, and may even be debatable. It certainly is not of prime importance to an appreciation of ethics, whatever one understands them (it) to be. Nonetheless, the confusion in verb number serves to illustrate another peculiarity: An explanation of ethics is difficult right from the start. In this respect it is similar to attempting an explanation of humor. The more one dissects it the more it loses impact.

The first reason for introducing the rather distressing situation of whether ethics is something-or-other, or ethics are something-or-other is first to dispel now any confusion that might exist as to whether the subject and verb do, or do not, agree. They always agree in this book, even when they look as if they don't. The second reason is to assist the reader in understanding the variety in verb number associated with the word ethics that appears throughout the text.

PROFESSIONAL ETHICS

Most dictionaries further describe the word *ethics* as being the study of standards of conduct and moral judgment; the system or code of morals of a particular person, religion, group, profession, and so forth. An ethic, then, is any singular element within a system of ethics.

Professional ethics is not a random collection of good behaviors; it is a **system** of conduct that is painstakingly developed to guide the practice of a specific discipline. Diane Hill, Ph.D. (1991), Corporate psychologist for Sommerville and Company, Inc., in Denver, describes ethics as the study of human conduct in light of specified moral principles. Other professionals suggest that ethical action is behavior consistent with society's security, order, and growth. Still others feel professional ethics is purely and simply The Golden Rule with a little added pizzazz.

The topic of ethics has grown to be one of the fundamental issues confronting modern society. The news media provide persistent notice of allegations and denials concerning corruption, fraud, influence peddling, institutional scandal, and substance abuse. Political impropriety and misbehavior in sports and religion make daily headlines. In varying degrees, all such reports impact principles on which human conduct is based. Although disturbed by these continuing revelations, it appears that the public has come to expect such occurrences as the standard behavior for government, business, and, increasingly, the professions.

THE EROSION OF PROFESSIONAL ETHICS

A look at the various professions today indicates that most have experienced an erosion of professional sovereignty as a result of demands that professional practitioners be more accountable to the consuming public. The traditional remoteness and paternalistic attitude of most professions are no longer acceptable to consumers, and consumerism, along with the information explosion, has curtailed people's willingness to continue the tradition of deferring passively to the judgments of professionals.

In the 1990s everybody wants to feel empowered. People demand to know what underlies the professionals' decisions. When clients or patients do second-guess professionals they are eager to question not only their competence, but their ethics as well. The misconduct that seemingly dominates the evening news has spawned a public perception that an appreciable number of professionals, physicians, lawyers, dentists, clergymen, politicians, and others unethically exploit their positions; and there is a growing common perception, as George Bernard Shaw (Veatch, 1982) put it, that "Every profession is a conspiracy against the laity."

Amid the public criticism of the professions it is in the best interest of every professional—beginning, intermediate, and experienced—to gain and regain an appreciation of what is expected of professionals within ethics.

Although it is difficult to recall a time when there was such pervasive skepticism about professional ethics, it is not difficult to recognize the present as an opportune time to change that wariness into a positive feeling toward the professions. In part this can be accomplished through education and a simple understanding that a profession[1] holds itself to a higher standard than the basic morals of the marketplace.

Unfortunately because of the dramatic rise in entrepreneurship, the once clear distinction between a business and a profession has become clouded. Unlike the decades before the 1960s, the opportunities for the professional practitioner are virtually unlimited. Today health care professionals can form publicly owned companies, obtain managed care contracts, secure venture capital, develop proprietary service-provider programs, dispense products, even make a profit—a word not usually used when speaking of the professions.

In many fields, however, there has been excessive profiteering—much to the dismay of the old-line professional. Traditionally alien in professions, that is now cause for alarm. In this upbeat, go-everywhere-fast society of the 1990s, far more so than in the era of the country Doc, the consumer is more apt to question the practitioner's motives for nearly every recommendation. To a large extent overuse of some medical treatments has resulted in the requirement by health insurance underwriters for a second opinion prior to approving payment for a surgical procedure, for example.

---

[1] *Profession* stems from the Latin **professio,** a public oath of fealty, or turning over one's loyalty to another.

In addition, it is an unavoidable fact that in some professions there are astonishingly high rates of reported misconduct. According to one survey (Pope & Bouhoutsos, 1986) between 8–12% of psychiatrists report having had sexual relations with their patients. As reported in the popular press there have been several thousand criminal indictments, civil monetary penalties, and settlements in cases of Medicare fraud and abuse. Major universities stand convicted in cases of fraud or misconduct in scientific research, authorship of scientific discovery, and allocation of research funds.

All these transgressions breach the system of ethics espoused by the professional organizations directly involved. Perusal of the case records buried in the law library of nearly any major university awaken one to many actual and potential violations of ethics in the professions.

Of course, there are far more practitioners who conform to society's expectations and who comply with their organization's system of ethical conduct than those who do not. It might be reasonable to wonder why attention is even directed toward the professions rather than, say, plumbers, TV repairmen, or used car sales people. One reason is clearly that professions traditionally command higher moral/ethical expectations than businesses or trades. A tradesman, for instance, is one who in ancient times literally trod the ground peddling wares from place-to-place. In modern times a tradesman, or a businessman, is no longer described as peddling wares, but is still viewed as predominantly associated with the marketplace.

In stark contrast, professionals of ancient times were practitioners who professed certain beliefs, who articulated *values* underlying their work. Today professionals continue to commit themselves to a set of values. The ethics of a business person are merely the morals of the marketplace, whereas the ethics of a professional is obedience to the principles and rules of conduct for an entire profession (Wright, 1987). Violations of these specified principles and rules usually result in some form of sanction imposed by the professional organization.

Fundamentally, professionals are distinguished from business people by three essential features (Resnick, 1991):

1. By achieving certification and/or licensure a professional obtains a special monopoly over the right to provide a social service. (This distinction does not accrue to business persons.)
2. Professionals have a defined scope of practice, deviations from which may violate the law. (A seller of carpets can suddenly shift and begin selling shoes, but an audiologist cannot suddenly start designing houses and be called an architect.)

3. Professionals comply with a clearly articulated set of values, or code of ethics. (Those who do not face sanction as severe as the loss of credentials necessary to engage in the practice of the profession.)

Despite these clear distinctions between business and profession there are individuals who resist any attempt to understand the ethics of professionalism and who continue to see no differences between the morals of the marketplace and the value standards of a profession. These individuals believe they are both a professional and a business person, and they believe their business ethics—do unto others—are equal to the system of ethics supported by professionals.

Although this may be true in isolated instances, it is neither presumptuous nor false to insist that the ethics of the two disciplines are motivated by different forces. As long as self-interest remains the driving force of business effort, the matter of professional ethics is excluded. This has to be so, because self-interest is not one of the stated values of any profession.

Professionals are committed to more than personal gain. Obviously professionals are paid for what they do, and it has been well stated by Pound (1953) that:

> Historically there are three ideas involved in a profession: organization, learning, i.e., pursuit of a learned art, and a spirit of public service. These are essential. A further idea, that of gaining a livelihood is involved in all callings. It is the main, if not the only purpose in the . . . money-making callings. In a profession it is incidental. (p. 87)

The relationship is a particularly troublesome concept for individuals who think of themselves as professionals and also as business persons. The issue is made more complex when the profession deals not only in service, but in products as well, as is the case with optometrists who sell eyeglasses, or audiologists who sell hearing aids.

Virtually all audiologists in private practice view themselves as professional/business individuals, primarily because they sell hearing aids. But even audiologists and speech-language pathologists in institutional settings are being required to manage departments as businesses as much as possible. Audiologists and speech-language pathologists can wrestle with the not-so-apparent difference between professional value standards and the morals of the marketplace for some time before they reach and feel comfortable with the balance that must exist between professional ethics and the reality of the business world.

The private practice of medicine traditionally has been and will continue to be both a profession and a business, but there has not been a great deal of confusion between the two areas in the past. However, in 1985 articles began to appear cautioning medical practitioners to be aware of the powerful economic incentives mounting to make the practice of medicine more of a business than ever.

Today these caveats are embellished by a spreading sense of doubt among physicians in general as to whether, in reality, the learned profession of medicine can be delivered into the next millennium as a true profession—not merely as a trade or business.

Medicine, dentistry, law, optometry, audiology, speech-language pathology, to mention a few, are *professions* first and foremost. Each has a defined scope of practice. Credentials are required to engage in the fields, and each subscribes to a stated set of values. Moreover, the practice of these professions is governed by a code of ethics, a set of rules guiding conduct of the practitioner and punishing proven deviations.

The private practice of each is also a business. But physicians, for example, are not noted for being business people. Although some are quite good at business economics, they are noted for practicing medicine. Highlighting that stature is not to ignore that physicians, dentists, lawyers, audiologists, and so forth, need to be concerned with the business matters of running an office. They do, as all professional practitioners do, but not to the exclusion of complying with their professional code of ethics. There is a harmony between business morals and professional ethics that must be achieved if professions are to survive in the traditional form.

In most states it is common practice for optometrists to dispense contact lenses. It is not as common, but certainly on the increase, for some ophthalmologists to prescribe and supply contact lenses to their patients. The procedure is still considered atypical of a medical specialty practice. Dispensing of hearing aids in an otolaryngology practice represents another atypical model.

It is reasonable for the ethics of such a dispensing situation to be questioned. The question focuses on the sale of a product by the one who prescribes it. Stated another way, there is an appearance of a conflict of interest when product sales are dependent on the prescription of the one who sells that specific product. Conflicts of interest do not always exist in such situations, thanks in part at least, to a code of ethics, but more will be said in the specific area of conflict of interest in Chapter 5. The overall danger that professional organizations face when their members become involved in product sales is that the practitioner, and thereby the organization, is at risk of becoming self-serving.

Most professional organizations today do not want to be self-serving; the groups want to serve society in ways that are consistent with order, security, and growth in health care provision. It is a safe assumption that professional practitioners want to continue to qualify for health insurance payments. No one wants to risk government curtailment of health services because of the apparent self-serving interests of practitioners.

PRESERVATION OF ETHICS

One might wonder how professional organizations can best provide a model to preserve the system of ethical standards of practice while aiding in the expansion of health care. Hill (1990) offers the five Ps of ethical leadership as useful in guiding the way not only to exhorting the members of a professional association to behaviors consistent with growth, order, and security in health care, but in preserving professional ethics within a practice. The attributes are: Purpose, Pride, Patience, Persistence, and Perspective. Performance might be added as a sixth consideration to Hill's list.

Purpose provides a roadmap that leads to consistency of direction within an association and within an individual. Purpose reduces ambiguity. Most importantly, it allows an organization or a person to march toward the full potential to affect change,rather than to just mark time.

Pride in one's organization and ethical behavior are reciprocal. Pride makes one want to do the right thing, and doing the right thing makes a person proud. Remember, it's managers who do things right. Leaders do the right thing. Pride sets the process in motion.

Patience is the third principle of ethical leadership. Being a listener, having the willingness to tolerate dissent, and being able to see ourselves as others see us pays dividends. It can provide the practitioners the ability to seek consumer suggestions to change, expand, and improve service.

Persistence, the fourth P of ethical leadership, emphasizes the theme that once goals and objectives of an association or a practice are identified, participants need to be encouraged to pursue them somewhat selfishly and not be influenced by outside pressures.

Perspective is the final concern on Hill's (1990) list. Perspective is easy to lose. The skill in maintaining perspective requires keeping priorities straight and maintaining a sense of how each practitioner fits into the overall picture. The hallmarks of perspective in leadership and organizations according to Hill (1990) are humor and manners.

Performance, of course, makes all the others work effectively and may be added to the list. Performance of one's professional duties, keeps not only the welfare of the consumer foremost, but also the image of the profession.

THE NORM OF RECIPROCITY

In addition to the six Ps, it is useful from the ethics standpoint to be aware of what social scientists refer to as the norm of reciprocity, or the obligation to help those who have helped you. The *norm of reciprocity* is one of the fundamental principles guiding human interactions. It is not surprising, therefore, that pharmaceutical companies (to mention one of many possible examples) rely on this principle of human nature by giving premiums to physicians in hopes they will prescribe their firms' products in return.

In the context of medicine, many U.S. senators are on the federal record as being opposed to the pharmaceutical practice, indicating that the act of accepting the gift has far-reaching ethical consequences that put the "gift" at too great a price. Numerous studies have attempted to determine the influence of pharmaceutical marketing practices on physician decision making. Unfortunately, the studies are problematic in that they rely on physician self-reporting, thus introducing a strong potential bias.

In an elegant study that to a large extent overcomes this problem, Jerry Avorn, M.D. (1982), associate professor of social medicine and health policy at Harvard Medical School, selects two classes of drugs with efficacy messages differing substantially between commercial and scientific sources.

The first class of medications, cerebral and peripheral vasodilators, were at the time widely promoted for the treatment of senile dementia and peripheral vascular insufficiency. The clinical literature indicated the products uselessness for both conditions.

The second class, propoxyphene products (especially Darvon®), were heavily promoted as effective relievers of moderately severe pain. The weight of scientific evidence suggested strongly that their analgesic properties were at best only equivalent to aspirin.

Avorn (1982) sampled a group of physicians regarding their beliefs about the drugs. Their responses were then used to determine the source of the physicians' information. Avorn writes:

> Although the vast majority of practitioners perceived themselves as paying little attention to drug advertisements and detail men [sic], as compared with papers in the scientific literature, their belief about effectiveness of the drugs revealed quite the opposite pattern of influence. This discrepancy could be caused by either (a) respondents' unwillingness to admit to reliance upon commercial sources, or (b) their lack of awareness of such influence. (p. 8)

Whatever the reasons, the point is clear that heavy marketing tactics have a positive commercial effect on those persons in a position of using, prescribing for use, buying, or making choices. The very nature of medical care provision is to make choices constantly. To decide to pursue a particular course of treatment is to decide that one is better than alternatives. To decide to fit a particular hearing aid or to continue with a specific dysphagia rehabilitation technique is to indicate that it is better than whatever the alternatives may be. Deciding that something is better than something else is to make a value judgment, and most of those judgments involve ethical choices.

Many value choices can be made instinctively. Not every value or ethical choice requires conscious thought—but in some cases intuition falters. What is needed is a system for ferreting out the issues involved and reflecting on the moral intuitions that underpin them, and, to the extent possible, eliminating or at least recognizing the temptations that erode quality choice-making.

Ethics is such a system of disciplined reflection on moral intuitions and moral choices. Ethics often begins with long-held beliefs and intuitions about something. Ethics attempts to compare beliefs and intuitions and draw inferences to develop rules of conduct about them and to articulate principles that might underlie the rules. At the end, ethics deals with what we mean when we say something is right or wrong. Increasingly ethics is being applied to real-world problems. It is an attractive system because it integrates rules and principles with knowledge of facts relevant to a particular sphere of life such as medicine, psychology, audiology, speech-language pathology, or even the total job environment. Professional ethics presents an especially attractive system, because it allows great emphasis to be placed on the giving of a service to humankind without the need for self-interest.

THE OATH OF HIPPOCRATES

There are a number of prominent positions in ethics as traditions, or bases for systems; but the most familiar, at least in Western civilization, is the Hippocratic tradition. The exact origin of the Hippocratic Oath is uncertain, but it probably came from one of the several different schools, or groups, of physicians who reflected different medical and philosophical beliefs. One of these schools emerged in the 5th century B.C. and produced a large quantity of scientific and ethical writings. The acknowledged head of the school was Hippocrates. Although he did not write all of the material that emanated from the group, Edelstein (1967) indicates the writings were gathered into collections known as the Hippocratic Corpus.

Although some of the writings describe human anatomy and deal with scientific problems, many are clearly ethical in theme. The writings include Precepts, Aphorisms, Law, On Decorum, and of course Oath. Oath is the shortest and by far the one of most historic interest. That is what is meant when one indicates that the foundation of ethics ascribed to Western physicians in the Hippocratic tradition has its roots in the Hippocratic Oath. The Oath is divided into two parts: the Pledge and the Code.

The Pledge

The first portion is an oath of allegiance. It pledges the Hippocratic physician to consider one's teacher as an equal to one's parents and to regard the teacher's offspring as equal to siblings. It also pledges the physician to share his knowledge only with those who have taken the Oath. That notion, according to historians, is consistent with the 4th century Greek society's concept of "secret groups" but inconsistent with the modern concept of sharing medical knowledge with the scientific community. The arrangement whereby the fledgling physician agrees to honor the teacher as a parent is, as described by writings of Etziony (1973), a pattern of 4th century Pythagoreans. The new initiate even agrees to help the teacher financially in time of need, according to the Oath.

The Code

The second part, referred to as the Code of Ethics, divides medicine into three areas: Dietetics, Pharmacology, and Surgery.

Dietetics

In the section on Dietetics the Hippocratic physician pledges to apply measures only for "the benefit of the sick according to my ability and judgment." This single thought is the one that most physicians carry with them as the essence of the Hippocratic ethic. Of course, it has been expanded to apply to all areas of medical patient management, and incorporates a message of do no harm, as well.

Pharmacology

In the section on Pharmacology the initiate pledges not to administer a deadly drug or give a woman an abortive remedy.

Surgery

In Surgery the Hippocratic physician pledges not to use the knife (that is, perform surgery) "even on sufferers from stone," (probably kidney), but [to] "withdraw in favor of such men as are engaged in this work." That portion of the pledge is not so much a vote in favor of referral to specialists as it is an expression of the Pythagorean view that surgery defiled their divine purity and it was thus better left to those who had no concern for ritual contamination. (Edelstein, 1967)

The remaining words in the Oath prohibit sexual relations with patients and enjoin confidentiality. The Oath ends by having the physician ask that if the Oath is kept, the practitioner be granted enjoyment of life and fame for all time to come, but that if it be broken, the opposite should be the individual's lot.

Because the Oath is a mixture of maxims and injunctions, it is not beyond criticism. Despite this, however, the Hippocratic Oath represents the summary of a physician's sense of ethical obligation.

OTHER BASES FOR ETHICS

The best example of a basis for comprehensive medical ethics in the Anglo-Saxon world, however, comes from John Gregory's (1817) "Lectures on the Duties and Qualifications of a Physician." At the very least, the obligation for the newly inducted physician to support a professor in time of financial need was excluded, being no longer regarded as a meaningful demonstration of a practitioner's ability to deserve the public trust. A great sigh of relief was probably heard from past and future Oath takers.

But the era's most influential development boosting ethical conduct in general was a by-product of an English hospital dispute in 1789. In that year an epidemic erupted, overburdening hospital staff and creating a bitter feud among physicians, surgeons, apothecaries, and nurses. The hospital's trustees approached a respected, retired physician, Thomas Percival, asking him to develop a scheme of professional conduct to eliminate future disputes. Percival's document (Percival, 1927) became the cornerstone of modern professional (medical) ethics. In many respects it is similar to the Hippocratic Oath, but there are important differences expanding the focus to the overall ethics of all health care, rather than just those aspects involving the physician giver of services. Percival's expression has greater social perspective than the Hippocratic Oath.

Percival communicated ethics beyond the medical community by suggesting that one who answers to a code of high values should unite compassion and stability, arrogance and control. Some half a century later the American Medical Association (AMA) developed its modern code of ethics based to a large degree on Percival's document. The AMA code was revised in 1903, 1912, 1947, and 1980, as society and the practice of medicine required.

Today there are many professional codes of ethics purporting to specify standardized ethical behavior for practitioners of a specific profession. Some remain in accord with the Hippocratic model; others have moved away from that paternalistic mode. The code of ethics of the American Nurses' Association (ANA) (American Nurses' Association, Committee on Ethics, 1979) for example, states in effect that respect for persons is the most fundamental principle. Of interest in the ANA code (1979) is the approach that **patients** "have the moral right to determine what will be done with their own person; to be given accurate information, . . . and to accept, refuse, or terminate treatment without coercion."

By contrast the American Pharmaceutical Association Code states, "a **pharmacist** should hold the health and safety of patients to be of first consideration," a considerably more dogmatic approach.

The wide variety of codes of ethics in professional arenas poses some interesting questions about the best way to use them. Often codes sound platitudinous because they express the wisdom of the group endorsing them and many times exclude the wishes of those who receive the services. Codes manage to express some very controversial ideas as well, at least questionable to those outside the professional group that endorses the code.

Some practitioners view the stipulations of a code as "law"; some as "guideposts." The Preamble to the 1980 revision of the American Medical Association code clearly states that the Principles are not laws, but are merely guides to responsible professional behavior.

Other codes of medical ethics have a far different status. The Nuremberg Code (World Medical Association, 1956), as an example, has the status of international law, and was motivated by the medical atrocities discovered during the Nuremberg trials following World War II. The Nuremberg Code became the first publicly produced code of ethics for a branch of medical practice. It displays a legal and a moral character quite different from professional codes generated by professional groups themselves.

The Nuremberg Code abandons the older notion that human subjects of research should be protected solely by the commitment of the professional and replaces it with a notion of self-determination for potential subjects, giving birth to the required informed consent.

The President's Commission on the Study of Ethical Problems in Medicine and Biomedical and Behavioral Research (1983) does not enjoy legally binding status, albeit the positions increasingly reflect the collective attitudes of the American public. In this document, as with the Nuremberg Code, it is difficult to discount the positions represented as having an ambiguous foundation.

Many differing formulations of a health professional's duty have been written by professional groups at different times and in varying places. Each does not always agree with another. The matter becomes even more complex when one realizes that professionals are not the only persons writing codes governing the practice of professions.

For instance, ethics has long been a matter of importance to religious groups. In fact most religious groups have codified positions on the ethics of medical decision making. Jewish scholars have long recognized that Judaism includes a set of laws that provides unique Jewish views on such matters as autopsy and abortion.

A Hebrew physician's oath is preserved from the 7th century as reported by Bleich (1979) and is referred to as the Oath of Asaf. It was administered to students by the teacher. In contrast to the Hippocratic Oath, there is a specific injunction to show mercy to the poor and the needy. There is also a warning to avoid sorcery, magic, and witchcraft.

Roman Catholic scholars have written on medical ethics problems since the Middle Ages (O'Rourke, 1986). Their viewpoint is from Christian theological ethics. Papal statements on abortion, contraception, and sexual ethics are widely circulated. Equally important, however, are their positions on other medical issues, including care of the terminally ill.

Protestant denominations have an endorsed official position on a broad range of medical ethical issues. Perhaps their most important contribution to ethics thinking is in their approach to medical ethical problems (Hauerwas, 1986). By tradition, Protestants are committed to allowing the lay person an increased role in ethical and theological matters. This is manifest in medical ethics with a heavy emphasis on the participation of lay persons in reaching decisions about their own care.

Thus the stipulations of ethical conduct for the professions sometimes have clear legal standing and function to determine what the law requires. In other cases codes are moral documents describing moral positions of members of a particular group. Among those codes viewed as moral codes, supporters expect members to treat such codes as guides to individual moral judgment. Other documents assume that members will follow them as moral rules of conduct in the best interests of those served professionally, and if they're ignored, negative reward may result.

ETHICS IN SOME NON-WESTERN CULTURES

Although the diversity of professional ethics is great within Western culture, it is even greater when a broader base is considered.

Practitioners who come from cultures outside the Anglo-American West often bring with them beliefs that are difficult to incorporate into the professional ethics systems of the West.

Islam

The ethics of the Islamic tradition are based on Quranic teaching (Rahman, 1981). The Oath of the Islamic Medical Association of the USA and Canada contains a prohibition on killing similar to that found in Jewish teachings. Islamic physicians are committed to the virtues of wisdom, strength, understanding, and fortitude. They are to be honest, modest, merciful, and objective.

China

In China evidence exists of medical ethical writings as early as Sun Szu-miao's 7th century (Unschuld, 1979) documentations. These writings, in contrast to many documents in Hippocratic medical ethics, are dependent on the major philosophical-ethical systems of the broader culture, in this case Buddhist influences. Confucian thought provides the basis for many other early Chinese medical ethics teachings. The classical virtues of Chinese professional ethics are humaneness, compassion, and filial piety. Filial piety is linked to a notion completely foreign to Hippocratic ethics.

India

The most important texts in ancient Indian medical ethics are the Caraka Samhita and the Caraka Susruta Samhita (Reich, 1978). The Caraka Samhita, written about the 1st century A.D., contains maxims appropriate to the elite Indian culture. The physician should lead the life of a celibate, speak only truth, grow hair and beard, eat no meat, carry no arms, and be free from envy. One of the earliest codes to address the problem of allocating health resources, the Caraka states, "No persons, who are hated by the king, or who are haters of the king or who are hated by the public, or who are haters of the public, shall receive treatment. Similarly, those who are extremely abnormal, wicked, . . . [miserable] . . . shall not receive treatment." Contrast that with the strong statements concerning the needy in the Judeo-Christian and Chinese ethics statements, and the silence on these matters in the Oath of Hippocrates.

The variety of concerns expressed by ethics codes is obviously great, and the attitudes of the formulators compared to the expectations of professions as well as lay persons affected by the codes is equally broad. In addition to codes are covenants and contracts and how these are perceived as guardian statements of professional practice.

CODES, COVENANTS, AND CONTRACTS

Not all professional ethical stipulations are in the form of codes. Some are position papers, essays written to defend a particular moral point of view or provide an analysis of several points of view—examination of euthanasia, for instance, or heart transplants for patients over the age of 70 are closer to position statements than principles and rules. Other ethics might be in the form of covenants or contracts. For an interesting and provocative analysis of this aspect of ethics the serious student is referred to William May (1975).

May examines the issue of ethics, covenants and contracts, and philanthropy from a realistic perspective. Basically he indicates that codes are patterns of behavior for particular groups and are especially relevant for inner circles within society. May expresses a feeling that codes tend to make conduct a matter of aesthetics, and sometimes they do so to the detriment of protecting objectivity within a profession. This is the case when public image becomes the prime motivator for having a code.

May contrasts a code as a means of articulating an ethic with a covenant. A covenant has historical roots which lead to a promissory event. The pledge that beginning physicians make to their teacher in the Hippocratic Oath is, then, a covenant. The obligations to patients the physician accepts in that same Oath is a code.

A contract, of course, involves at least two parties in a legally binding situation wherein they negotiate their own best interest and agree on some best means of deriving that interest to the benefit of each. The sale of a car, for example, is done by contractual arrangement whereby one party expresses an amount offered for the vehicle and the second party accepts the amount in exchange for the car under certain conditions of payment and so forth.

That use of the contract concept is quite rigid for application to applied ethics, however. The term "social contract" is perhaps better. Social contract implies that members of a given society agree on what the principles of the society should be and try as a group to uphold them. Penalties come into play when the principles are not upheld. Here is where the whole matter of ethics becomes difficult. Some (usually the violators) say that the principles are only guides. Some (the ethicists who framed the code) say that the principles are the "law."

Different views of ethics have been held by different groups during varying periods of history. The predominant and persistent view has been that only persons with special skills, knowledge, or training can know and appreciate ethical truths. This, in fact, is the position of the Hippocratic tradition. It is controversial in modern society, one that most have modified to support the position that everyone, not just a select few, has moral insight. That position is based on the belief that morality, even if ethics is more than just morality, is universal in the sense that a common set of principles applies across the board to all living things. Morality is something everybody knows. It does not need requisite special esoteric skills.

Be all that as it may, society at least for now continues to demand accountability and trust, and professions abide by the tradition of a code of ethics as the best means of demonstrating these traits to the public. Change in the understanding of ethics is inevitable, and it is good. What is crucial to preserving professional ethics as a viable system, however, is the need for practitioners of health professions to recognize what they have at present as a means to sustain the public confidence in their services. Once there is recognition, the question becomes whether to preserve the distinctive quality of a profession over and above, and separate from, the quality of a business.

The ethics of businesses is different from the ethics of professions. For one thing business ethics has no scholarly or traceable history. For another, scholars, philosophers, religious leaders, ethicists, and so forth do not debate the issue of business ethics. Business ethics change to fit the marketplace. They may change hourly, daily, from town to town, and from businessperson to businessperson.

There are those who believe that no profession exists for itself; that each exists for a purpose and that purpose will be increasingly defined by society. Whatever the rationale for existence of a profession proves to be in the 21st century, a system of values in which self-interest is clearly incidental is fundamental to any. And that system is a code of ethics.

2

The Code of Ethics

A society without any objective legal scale is a terrible one indeed. I know; I have lived in one. But a society with no scale but the legal one is not quite worthy of man either. (Alexander Solzhenitzyn)

Many people believe a code of ethics to be a document specific only to professional organizations such as the American Medical Association (AMA), American Psychological Association (APA), the American Bar Association (ABA), or the American Speech-Language-Hearing Association (ASHA), and so on. The perception is not correct. Trade associations, unions, and even businesses can, and sometimes do, develop a code of ethics. Usually the codes of trades and businesses do not compare to any significant degree to the expressions and intents embodied in professional codes of ethics, however. The fundamental difference is in the caliber of values expressed by each. Most ethics codes are found among professional organizations, rather than trades or businesses, because professional organizations are built on values which hold foremost the interests of people served.

WHAT ARE ETHICS CODES?

There is nothing mysterious about a code of ethics, nor is there anything particularly exclusive about it except for its support of an organization's principles. A code of ethics is most often nothing more than a series of statements setting forth the values of an organization through a listing of its principles (Konold, 1978). The principles are achieved when practitioners of the profession comply with a set of rules that provide the minimum standards and behavioral expectations necessary to support the principles.

Equally important to the professional code of ethics is that it traditionally carries with it an array of sanctions, or punishments, to be meted out for proven violations of the code. Sanctions can range from a confidential reprimand issued by a monitoring committee or board, to revocation of credentials necessary to the practice of the specific profession. The code is generally under the control of a committee, or board of peers, selected from the membership of the professional association they represent. Among the many obligations of a professional association is the responsibility to revise the code as changes in the provision of a service may require (Titus & Keeton, 1978). The benefits that an organization reaps from a code are, at the very least, an enhancement of public stature and a general homogeneity to the practice of the profession represented by the document. Credibility of, and accountability for, the services provided by the professional association are also substantial benefits.

Codes of professional ethics haven't changed much in intent over the years, although content and emphasis has shifted periodically in some professions to reflect societal changes and interpretations (King, 1982). Physicians have been seen as professionals in the traditional sense as having both a body of specialized knowledge and a commitment to a distinctive ethic binding them to special norms, unique duties, and higher values, according to the British Medical Association (1984). Physicians, for whatever reason, have always had a very special code of ethics, which is emulated in many aspects by codes of other professions.

Fundamentally all codes are group-inspired documents, painstakingly prepared, that appear in a variety of forms and, today, for a multitude of reasons. Most commonly, codes govern professional conduct and protect professional interests. The most customary shared trait among them is that the documents attempt to control the practice behavior of the professional. There is little apparent regard in most codes that consumers of professional service may also have minds capable of participating in some aspects of their care, or that the provider of services may in some instances need to adjust practice standards to meet special circumstances. There are few exceptions.

Some codes inspire, or even set, high standards for practitioners. Others guide research or clarify contractual agreements. Some codes describe duties and obligations to those served, to colleagues, and to associates. All codes uphold the honor and tradition of the profession that authors them. They serve as a foundation for professional pride.

Vollmer and Mills (1966) indicate that ethical codes per se are more often associated with the most highly professionalized occupations. They also relate that trade occupations bent on upgrading their status deliberately explored the introduction of formal ethical codes in the belief that such public statements would not only engender greater occupational conformity, but also bring about more public support and respect.

In 1992, despite those efforts, there is still a greater number of codes of ethics among the traditional professions than any other occupation. The fact remains, nonetheless, that most often a code of ethics is developed by an organization for two (sometimes three) purposes:

1. To improve/preserve the behavior of organization members,
2. To improve/protect public perception of the organization, and agreeing to abide by the code of ethics *may*, in some cases,
3. Provide the basis for membership in the organization.

At the first official meeting of the American Medical Association (AMA) in 1847, one of the initial important items of business was the establishment of a code of ethics, which was used as a guide to professional practice (American Medical Association, 1848). In 1848, a Committee on Ethics (now the Council on Ethical and Judicial Affairs) of the AMA was appointed to interpret and implement the ethics code. The Code of Ethics of the American Medical Association (1981) has been recognized as an authoritative source of medical ethics by physicians, courts, legislatures, and medical licensing boards since its inception.

The code has provided physicians with guidance on a full range of ethics questions, from genetic engineering, to euthanasia, to organ donation. In 1868, for example, the AMA through its Council on Ethical and Judicial Affairs urged that women be entitled to practice medicine. More recently the association has issued path-breaking opinions on the physicians' obligation to treat patients with AIDS, or other HIV infections.

The AMA's Code of Ethics (1984) consists of three integrated components: The Principles of Medical Ethics, the Current Opinions of the Council on Ethical and Judicial Affairs, and Reports of the Council on Ethical and Judicial Affairs. The Principles of Medical Ethics are seven precepts that broadly define the ethical boundaries of medical practice. Applications of the Principles to specific ethical issues in the practice of medicine constitute the Current Opinions. Reports detail in written form the consideration and reasoning of the Council in reaching conclusions on matters involving ethical questions.

The cornerstone of the AMA Code is, of course, the seven Principles. Inspired by the Oath of Hippocrates and revised by subsequent statements of physicians' professional responsibilities over the years, the Principles recognize the practitioners' obligations to patients, the profession, and to society. They provide solid foundation for the public trust afforded the learned profession of medicine. Ethicists in modern times, however, point out that there is an obligation for the principles to at least recognize the rights of those persons served professionally. It is that recognition that gave motion to bioethics thinking and added the rights and wishes of persons on whom service was being imposed to the equation.

ADVANTAGES OF ETHICS CODES

Virtually all ethics codes enhance the profession that supports them in several areas, such as educating members, introducing norms for new members to aspire to, providing information to the consumer, deterring bad conduct, disciplining offenders, and, of course, protecting the public (Stromberg, 1990).

For example, in the area of **education** ethics codes help to inform all members of the profession—particularly younger members entering the field. Through a listing of principles and rules in the code, for instance, the values and standards of practice of the group, all members are presented with a constant and consistent benchmark of performance. Members learn the standards of practice in a given profession by conformity.

Codes encourage members, new as well as old, to aspire to the very highest levels of conduct expressed as principles. The principles included in a professional code of ethics can be thought of as the **aspirational norms** of professional practice. Even though it may not be unethical to fall below the stated principles, most members will attempt to achieve the highest standard by complying with, or exceeding, the rules expressed under each principle. Failure to comply with the rules of a code of ethics, however, may result in penalty to the violator. All professional organizations distinguish, in one way or another, between principles (to aspire to) and rules (noncompliance with which may trigger sanction).

Codes **provide information to consumers**. Today, most applications for professional positions, research grants, staff privileges, faculty positions, etc. require that the applicant disclose episodes of misconduct that are a matter of record. Findings of misconduct, for example, sanctioned violations of the code of ethics of an organization, are often published in journals, professional newsletters, and so forth. In some professions, and audiology and speech-language pathology are two of them, prestigious credentials that have taken years to acquire can be revoked for violations of the code. In this manner the ethics process provides meaningful information to the marketplace that can assist the consumer of direct services, in addition to those who function as referral sources, to make informed comparisons about the qualifications of professionals.

A believable and defensible code of ethics monitored by an informed and strong Ethical Practice Board usually serves effectively to **deter bad conduct** before it occurs. Often a letter to a practitioner from the Ethical Practice Board suggesting that a potential for unethical conduct exists in some aspect of the particular practice goes a long way toward avoiding actual citation.

Obviously, a central goal of a viable professional code of ethics is to assure the quality of service provided by practitioners. This may be accomplished by imposing sanctions on those who fail to meet the rules of the Code—that is, **by disciplining offenders**. The effectiveness of sanctions depends to a great extent on the economics of the profession. In such fields as law, medicine, and even audiology and speech-language pathology, in which referrals and professional affiliations are of great importance, being branded as unethical can have serious economic impact.

Naturally, along with enhancing the image of the profession, guarding the consumer against less-than-quality service is the primary reason for having a code of ethics. Well worded codes **protect the public**.

Unfortunately, codes represent only a single step in protecting users of professional service against charlatanism, fraud, deception, and so forth, as well as achieving the other spin-off benefits for the association. No code of ethics can *ensure* the complete protection of the public, or attainment of any of the ancillary goals.

CONSIDERATIONS IN DEVELOPING A CODE

The development of a code of ethics is a difficult, sometimes agonizing task fraught with difficult little problems. Realizing that developers of a code may also be practitioners of the profession one can presume that a degree of self-preservation is usually present when a group meets to develop a code of ethics. Therefore, great care must be taken to assure that the language of the code reflects the values of the profession and not the biases of a group within it.

Recall that the entire code of ethics of the AMA consists of seven statements of principles. It is the interpretations later formulated by the AMA's Committee on Ethical and Judicial Affairs as questions regarding the principles arise that are the working tools of the Code. Some associations believe this to be the preferred way of developing a code of ethics. Others feel that it fails to provide early guidance to members.

Selection of the language itself is demanding. On the one hand, a code cannot be written in such legalistic terms that every alleged violation becomes a case for the courts to decide. On the other hand, neither can the principles and rules be expressed in such broad terms as to be unmeasurable, or for that matter, unachievable. Additionally, some people feel that a code should be concise and not attempt to provide for every possible ethics transgression. In such a case the stated principles become the important aspects, and, as deviations are reported, interpretations are published, which then form the standards of practice. The oldest code, that of the AMA, follows this paradigm.

A CODE OF ETHICS

The Code of Ethics of the American Academy of Audiology (AAA) was adopted in the fall of 1990 and published in January 1991. At the time this chapter was written it was the newest professional Code of Ethics published by a professional organization. It consists of two parts: a Statement of Principles and Rules (American Academy of Audiology, 1991) and the Procedures.

Part I of the Code, Statement of Principles and Rules, is reproduced here to stimulate thinking by the reader on the professional value statements that serve the purposes of the code. Comments and questions are enclosed in brackets following many of the Principles and Rules. They are meant to be representative of the kinds of concerns held by formulators of ethics codes and the author of this book takes full responsibility for their content. The comments are not to be considered as part of the code text. By including the code as part of the text, rather than as an Appendix, reference to it easily can be made while reading the chapter.

Although the code consists of two parts, Part II provides the processes that enable enforcement of the Principles and Rules. It has been omitted from the chapter because the procedures organizations develop reflect the process needs of those organizations and have no societal implications. In that they are strictly mechanical, they have little application to the discussion of ethics.

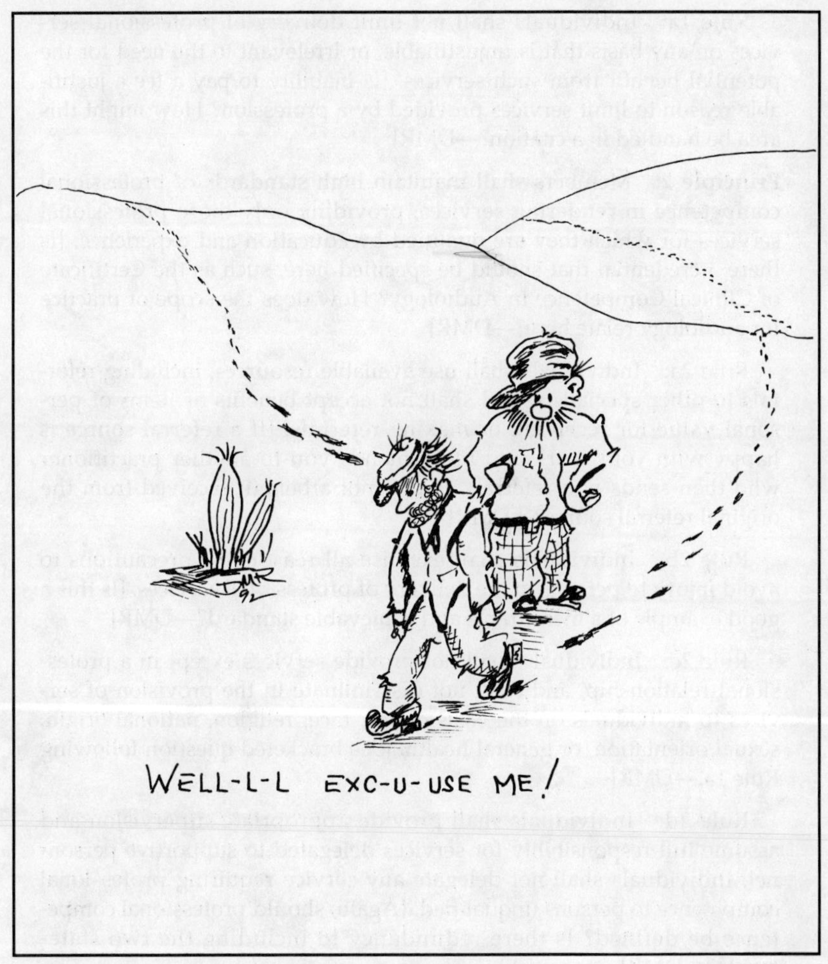

Following the presentation of the American Academy of Audiology Code, the 1991 Code of Ethics of the American Speech-Language-Hearing Association is given for comparative purposes and further discussion.

American Academy of Audiology
Code of Ethics (Jan. 1991)

Part I

Principle 1: Members shall provide professional services with honesty and compassion and shall respect the dignity, worth and rights of those served.

Rule 1a: Individuals shall not limit delivery of professional services on any basis that is unjustifiable, or irrelevant to the need for the potential benefit from such services. [Is inability to pay a fee a justifiable reason to limit services provided by a profession? How might this area be handled in a citation?—DMR]

Principle 2:   Members shall maintain high standards of professional competence in rendering services, providing only those professional services for which they are qualified by education and experience. [Is there a credential that should be specified here, such as the Certificate of Clinical Competence in Audiology? How does the scope of practice for audiology relate here?—DMR]

Rule 2a: Individuals shall use available resources, including referrals to other specialists, and shall not accept benefits or items of personal value for receiving or making referrals. [If a referral source is happy with your work and recommends you to another practitioner who then sends you referrals, is that not a benefit received from the original referral source?—DMR]

Rule 2b: Individuals shall exercise all reasonable precautions to avoid injury to persons in the delivery of professional services. [Is this a good example of a measurable and achievable standard?—DMR]

Rule 2c: Individuals shall not provide services except in a professional relationship, and shall not discriminate in the provision of services to individuals on the basis of sex, race, religion, national origin, sexual orientation, or general health. [See bracketed question following Rule 1a.—DMR]

Rule 2d: Individuals shall provide appropriate supervision and assume full responsibility for services delegated to supportive personnel. Individuals shall not delegate any service requiring professional competence to persons unqualified. [Again, should professional competence be defined? Is there redundancy to including the two statements?—DMR]

Rule 2e: Individuals shall not permit any person to engage in any practice that is a violation of the Code of Ethics.

Rule 2f: Individuals shall maintain professional competence, including participation in continuing education. [Should some amount of time be specified such as at least once a year?—DMR]

Principle 3:   Members shall maintain the confidentiality of the information and records of those receiving services. [What about the records of those who have already received services?—DMR]

Rule 3a: Individuals shall not reveal to any unauthorized persons any professional or personal information obtained from the person served professionally, unless required by law.

Principle 4: Members shall provide only services and products that are in the best interest of those served.

Rule 4a: Individuals shall not exploit persons in the delivery of professional services. [Should "products" be included?—DMR]

Rule 4b: Individuals shall charge only for services rendered. [Does this preclude the practice of charging for appointments missed and not canceled?—DMR]

Rule 4c: Individuals shall not participate in activities that constitute a conflict of professional interest. [Is it important to include "or the appearance of conflict of interest"?—DMR]

Rule 4d: Individuals shall not accept compensation for supervision or sponsorship beyond reimbursement of expenses. [Because of this wording, are people employed as supervisors at risk of violating the code?—DMR]

Principle 5:   Members shall provide accurate information about the nature and management of communicative disorders and about the services and products offered. [By whose definition is "accurate information" judged?—DMR]

Rule 5a: Individuals shall provide the persons served with the information a reasonable person would want to know about the nature and possible effects of services rendered, or products provided.

Rule 5b: Individuals may make a statement of prognosis, but shall not guarantee results, mislead, or misinform persons served.

Rule 5c: Individuals shall not carry out teaching or research activities in a manner that constitutes an invasion of privacy or that fails to inform persons fully about the nature and possible effects of these activities, affording all persons informed free-choice and participation.

Rule 5d: Individuals shall maintain documentation of professional services rendered. [Is it important to specify a time period?—DMR]

Principle 6:   Members shall comply with the ethical standards of the Academy with regard to public statements.

Rule 6a: Individuals shall not misrepresent their educational degrees, training, credentials, or competence. Only degrees earned from regionally accredited institutions in which training was obtained in audiology, or a directly related discipline, may be used in public statements concerning professional services. [Should "misrepresent" be defined?—DMR]

Rule 6b: Individuals' public statements about professional services and products shall not contain representations or claims that are false, misleading, or deceptive.

Principle 7: Members shall honor their responsibilities to the public and to professional colleagues.

Rule 7a: Individuals shall not use professional or commercial affiliations in any way that would mislead or limit services to persons served professionally. [Are there antitrust implications in this statement?—DMR]

Rule 7b: Individuals shall inform colleagues and the public in a manner consistent with the highest professional standards about products and services they have developed.

Principle 8: Members shall uphold the dignity of the profession and freely accept the Academy's self-imposed standards.

Rule 8a: Individuals shall not violate these Principles and Rules, nor attempt to circumvent them.

Rule 8b: Individuals shall not engage in dishonesty or illegal conduct that adversely reflects on the profession. [How about *legal* conduct that adversely reflects on the profession?—DMR]

Rule 8c: Individuals shall inform the Ethical Practice Board when there are reasons to believe that a member of the Academy may have violated the Code of Ethics. [Is failure to inform, then, a violation of the Code?—DMR]

Rule 8d: Individuals shall cooperate with the Ethical Practice Board in any matter related to the Code of Ethics.

ANOTHER CODE OF ETHICS

Ethics codes of other professions can be looked at in similar fashion. For example, the Code of Ethics of the American Speech-Language-Hearing Association (1991), revised January 1991, specifies the fundamental rules of ethical conduct in three categories designated as Principles of Ethics, Ethical Proscriptions, and Matters of Professional Propriety. A Preamble to the ASHA Code describes each of these areas.

Principles and Proscriptions

Five Principles serve as the basis for evaluation of professional conduct from an ethics viewpoint in the ASHA Code of Ethics. These Principles form the underlying moral basis of the Code and are to be observed by members of the Association under all conditions of professional activity.

Ethical Proscriptions are presented in the 1991 ASHA Code as formal statements of prohibitions that are derived from the stated Principles of Ethics.

Matters of Professional Propriety

Matters of Professional Propriety, as described in the Preamble to the ASHA Code, represent guidelines of conduct designed to promote the public trust and inform consumers about the services available and the rules that govern the provision of those services.

DISCUSSION OF THE ASHA CODE

The 1991 version of the Code also consists of 5 well-worded Principles of Ethics (some listing subprinciples as well, which are 11 in number), 18 Ethical Proscriptions, and 8 Matters of Professional Propriety. The process of filing complaints, Board procedures, and sanctions is not part of the ASHA Code of Ethics.

For the most part, the document is a good example of what a Code should be, although it has been criticized, when small groups convene, as being paternalistic. The technique of separating the aspirations and guidelines into three categories is an interesting, but not common, way of presenting a code of ethics. Perhaps because of the size of the American Speech-Language-Hearing Association (about 65,000 in 1991) and the interest of its members in the private practice of their profession, attention to updates and revisions in the code is keen. In some areas of practice the standard has changed so drastically that it is the **Code** that is clearly not reflective of current standards of practice. An example is dispensing hearing aids to the consumer by audiologists, a practice not in compliance with the 1991 ASHA Code, but a standard practice among many audiologists since the late 1970s.

The ASHA maintains not only an Ethical Practices Board to monitor the conduct of member practitioners, but also a Council on Professional Ethics. The council functions both to revise the Code and as an appeals body, as well as to monitor and set the standards of the association, among other things.

The 1991 version of the ASHA Code of Ethics document is presented for comparison with the Code of the American Academy of Audiology on style and overall content. The intent of the presentations in this chapter is not to be critical of either document, but rather to instruct by comparing two ethics codes.

A 1992 revision of the ASHA Code follows the reprint of the 1991 edition.

The most apparent difference to be noted between the AAA and ASHA codes is that the ASHA 1991 version appears lengthy and is often redundant. There is a lack of balance between Ethical Proscriptions and Matters of Professional Propriety in the ASHA Code, although balance is not a characteristic of most codes. Is it reasonable to include, for instance, more Matters of Professional Propriety than Ethical Proscriptions? Look also at each statement to determine whether (1) it will be possible to measure behavior against the proscriptions sufficiently to cite a violation, and (2) the conduct described is achievable. Recognize, too, that many of the questions posed for the American Academy of Audiology Code of Ethics also apply to the following code.

Code of Ethics of the American Speech-Language-Hearing Association
(revised January 1991)

PREAMBLE

The preservation of the highest standards of integrity and ethical principles is vital to the discharge of the professional responsibilities of all speech-language pathologists and audiologists. This Code of Ethics has been promulgated by the Association in an effort to stress the fundamental rules considered essential to the basic purpose. Any action that is a violation of the spirit and purpose of this Code shall be considered unethical. Failure to specify any particular responsibility or practice in the Code of Ethics should not be construed as denial of the existence of other responsibilities or practices.

The fundamental rules of ethical conduct are described in three categories: Principles of Ethics, Ethical Proscriptions, Matters of Professional Propriety.

1. Principles of Ethics. Five principles serve as a basis for the ethical evaluation of professional conduct and form the underlying moral basis for the Code of Ethics. Individuals subscribing to this Code shall observe these principles as affirmative obligations under all conditions of professional activity.

2. Ethical Proscriptions. Ethical proscriptions are formal statements of prohibitions that are derived from the Principles of Ethics.

3. Matters of Professional Propriety. Matters of Professional Propriety represent guidelines of conduct designed to promote the public interest and thereby better inform the public, and particularly the persons in need of speech-language pathology and audiology services as to the availability and the rules regarding the delivery of those services.

PRINCIPLE OF ETHICS I

Individuals shall hold paramount the welfare of persons served professionally.

A. Individuals shall use every resource available, including referral to other specialists as needed, to provide the best service possible.

B. Individuals shall fully inform persons served of the nature and possible effects of services.

C. Individuals shall fully inform subjects participating in research or teaching activities of the nature and possible effects of these activities.

D. Individuals' fees shall be commensurate with services rendered. [How would a violation be shown?—DMR]

E. Individuals shall provide appropriate access to records of persons served professionally.

F. Individuals shall take all reasonable precautions to avoid injuring persons in the delivery of services.

G. Individuals shall evaluate services rendered and products dispensed to determine effectiveness. [How is this to be done?—DMR]

Ethical Proscriptions

1. Individuals must not exploit persons in the delivery of professional services, including accepting persons for treatment when benefit cannot reasonably be expected, or continuing treatment unnecessarily.

2. Individuals must not guarantee the results of any therapeutic procedures directly or by implication. A reasonable statement of prognosis may be made but caution must be exercised not to mislead persons served professionally to expect results that cannot be predicted from sound evidence.

3. Individuals must not use persons for teaching or research in a manner that constitutes an invasion of privacy or fails to involve informed free choice to participate.

4. Individuals must not evaluate or treat speech, language, or hearing disorders except in a professional relationship. They must not evaluate or treat solely by correspondence. This does not preclude follow-up correspondence with persons previously seen, nor providing them with general information of an educational nature.

5. Individuals must not reveal to unauthorized persons any professional or personal information obtained from the person served professionally, unless required by law or unless necessary to protect the welfare of the person or the community.

6. Individuals must not discriminate in the delivery of professional services on any basis that is unjustifiable or irrelevant to the need for and potential benefit from such services, such as race, sex, age, religion, national origin, sexual orientation, or handicapping condition.

7. Individuals must not charge for services not rendered. [What are ethical implications of charging for missed appointments?—DMR]

PRINCIPLE OF ETHICS II

Individual shall maintain high standards of professional competence.

A. Individuals engaging in clinical practice or supervision thereof shall hold the appropriate Certificate(s) of Clinical Competence for the area(s) in which they are providing or supervising professional services.

B. Individuals shall continue their professional development throughout their professional careers.

C. Individual shall identify competent, dependable referral sources for persons served professionally.

D. Individuals shall maintain adequate records of professional services rendered.

Ethical Proscriptions

1. Individuals must neither provide service nor supervision of services for which they have not been properly prepared, nor permit services to be provided by any of their staff who are not properly prepared.

2. Individuals must not provide clinical services by prescription of anyone who does not hold the Certificate of Clinical Competence. [Are physicians who write prescriptive orders exempted?—DMR]

3. Individuals must not delegate any service requiring the professional competence of a certified clinician to anyone unqualified. [Is a Clinical Fellow or a student in training exempted?—DMR]

4. Individuals must not offer clinical services by supportive personnel, students, or clinical fellows for whom they do not provide appropriate supervision and assume full responsibility. [Does this cancel the previous rule?—DMR]

5. Individuals must not require anyone under their supervision to engage in any practice that is a violation of the Code of Ethics. [Should there be some reference to students in training being an exception?—DMR]

PRINCIPLE OF ETHICS III

Individuals' statements to persons served professionally and to the public shall provide accurate information about the nature and management of communicative disorders, and about the profession and services rendered by its practitioners.

Ethical Proscriptions

1. Individuals must not misrepresent their training or competence. [How should this be defined?—DMR]

2. Individuals' public statements providing information about professional services and products must not contain misrepresentations or claims that are false, deceptive, or misleading.

3. Individuals must not use professional or commercial affiliations in any way that would mislead or limit services to persons served professionally.

Matters of Professional Propriety

4. Individuals should announce services in a manner consonant with highest professional standards in the community.

PRINCIPLE OF ETHICS IV

Individuals shall honor their responsibilities to the public, their profession, and their relationships with colleagues and members of allied professions.

Ethical Proscriptions

1. Individuals must not participate in activities that constitute a conflict of professional interest. [How should "conflict of interest" be described?—DMR]

Matters of Professional Propriety

2. Individuals should seek to provide and expand services to persons with speech, language and hearing handicaps as well as to assist in establishing high professional standards for those programs.

3. Individuals should educate the public about speech, language, and hearing processes, speech, language, and hearing problems, and matters related to professional competence.

4. Individuals should strive to increase knowledge within the profession and share research with colleagues.

5. Individuals should establish harmonious relations with colleagues and members of other professions, and endeavor to inform members of related professions of services provided by speech-language pathologists and audiologists, as well as seek information from them.

6. Individuals should assign credit to those who have contributed to a publication in proportion to their contribution.

7. Individuals should not accept compensation for supervision or sponsorship from the clinical fellow being supervised or sponsored beyond reasonable reimbursement for direct expenses.

8. Individuals should present products they have developed to their colleagues in a manner consonant with highest professional standards.

PRINCIPLE OF ETHICS V

Individuals shall uphold the dignity of the profession and freely accept the profession's self-imposed standards.

A. Individuals shall inform the Ethical Practice Board when they have reason to believe that a member or certificate holder may have violated the Code of Ethics.

B. Individuals shall cooperate fully with the Ethical Practice Board concerning matters of professional conduct related to this Code of Ethics.

Ethical Proscriptions

1. Individuals shall not engage in violations of the Principles of Ethics or in any attempt to circumvent them.

2. Individuals shall not engage in dishonesty, fraud, deceit, misrepresentation, or other forms of illegal conduct that adversely reflects on the profession or the individual's fitness for membership in the profession.

During 1991, ASHA revised its Code of Ethics and the revision received approval of the Legislative Council in November of that year to become effective in January 1992. It is unusual for an organization to revise a Code of Ethics after only one year unless there are gross oversights. Obviously, the approval for audiologists to dispense hearing aids was of great concern to the stated ethics of the Association since the 1991 version did not permit hearing aid dispensing as an ethical practice. Because most audiologists today dispense hearing aids, that change was clearly necessary. In your reading the revised (1992) version try to find other reasons for the changes. The revisions are not indiscriminate. They are modifications that represent the reasoned thinking of professionals involved in the practice of the disciplines addressed by the document. The most recent revision (ASHA, 1992) follows:

Code of Ethics of the American Speech-Language-Hearing Association
(Revised January 1992)

PRINCIPLE OF ETHICS I

Individuals shall honor their responsibility to hold paramount the welfare of persons they serve professionally.

Rules of Ethics

A. Individuals shall provide all services competently.

B. Individuals shall use every resource, including referral when appropriate, to ensure that high-quality service is provided.

C. Individuals shall not discriminate in the delivery of professional services on the basis of race, sex, age, religion, national origin, disability or sexual orientation.

D. Individuals shall fully inform the persons they serve of the nature and possible effects of services rendered and products dispensed.

E. Individuals shall evaluate the effectiveness of services rendered and of products dispensed and shall provide services or dispense products only when benefit can reasonably be expected.

F. Individuals shall not guarantee the results of any treatment or procedure, directly or by implication; however, they may make a reasonable statement of prognosis.

G. Individuals shall not treat speech, language, or hearing disorders solely by correspondence.

H. Individuals shall maintain adequate records of professional services rendered and products dispensed and shall allow access to these records when appropriately authorized.

I. Individuals shall not reveal, without authorization, any professional or personal information about the person served professionally, unless required by law to do so, or unless doing so is necessary to protect the welfare of the person or of the community.

J. Individuals shall not charge for services not rendered, nor shall they misrepresent[1], in any fashion, services rendered or products dispensed.

K. Individuals shall use persons in research or as subjects of teaching demonstrations only with their informed consent.

L. Individuals shall withdraw from professional practice when substance abuse or an emotional or mental disability may adversely affect the quality of services they render.

PRINCIPLE OF ETHICS II

Individuals shall honor their responsibility to achieve and maintain the highest level of professional competence.

---

[1] For purposes of this Code of Ethics, misrepresentation includes any untrue statements or statements that are likely to mislead. Misrepresentation also includes the failure to state any information that is material and that ought, in fairness, to be considered.

Rules of Ethics

A. Individuals shall engage in the provision of clinical services only when they hold the appropriate Certificate of Clinical Competence or when they are in the certification process and are supervised by an individual who holds the appropriate Certificate of Clinical Competence.

B. Individuals shall engage in only those aspects of the professions that are within the scope of their competence, considering their level of education, training, and experience.

C. Individuals shall continue their professional development throughout their careers.

D. Individuals shall delegate the provision of clinical services only to persons who are certified or to persons in the education or certification process who are appropriately supervised. The provision of support services may be delegated to persons who are neither certified nor in the certification process only when a certificate holder provides appropriate supervision.

E. Individuals shall prohibit any of their professional staff from providingservices that exceed the staff member's competence, considering the staff member's level of education, training, and experience.

F. Individuals shall ensure that all equipment used in the provision of services is in proper working order and is properly calibrated.

PRINCIPLE OF ETHICS III

Individuals shall honor their responsibility to the public by promoting public understanding of the professions, by supporting the development of services designed to fulfill the unmet needs of the public, and by providing accurate information in all communications involving any aspect of the professions.

Rules of Ethics

A. Individuals shall not misrepresent their credentials, competence, education, training, or experience.

B. Individuals shall not participate in professional activities that constitute a conflict of interest.

C. Individuals shall not misrepresent diagnostic information, services rendered, or products dispensed or engage in any scheme or artifice to defraud in connection with obtaining payment or reimbursement for such services or products.

D. Individuals' statements to the public shall provide accurate information about the nature and management of communication disorders, about the professions, and about professional services.

E. Individuals' statements to the public—advertising, announcing and marketing their professional services, reporting research results, and promoting products—shall adhere to prevailing professional standards and shall not contain misrepresentations.

PRINCIPLE OF ETHICS IV

Individuals shall honor their responsibilities to the professions and their relationships with colleagues, students, and members of allied professions. Individuals shall uphold the dignity and autonomy of the professions, maintain harmonious interprofessional and intraprofessional relationships, and accept the professions' self-imposed standards.

Rules of Ethics

A. Individuals shall prohibit any staff under their supervision from engaging in any practice that violates the Code of Ethics.

B. Individuals shall not engage in dishonesty, fraud, deceit, misrepresentation, or any form of conduct that adversely reflects on the professions or on the individual's fitness to serve persons professionally.

C. Individuals shall assign credit only to those who have contributed to a publication, presentation, or product. Credit shall be assigned in proportion to the contribution and only with the contributor's consent.

D. Individuals' statements to colleagues about professional services, research results, and products shall adhere to prevailing professional standards and shall contain no misrepresentation.

E. Individuals shall not provide professional services without exercising independent professional judgment, regardless of referral source or prescription.

F. Individuals who have reason to believe that the Code of Ethics has been violated shall inform the Ethical Practice Board.

G. Individuals shall cooperate fully with the Ethical Practice Board in its investigation and adjudication of matters related to this Code of Ethics.

There are several features about this new Code that differ from the 1991 version. First, the document is reduced to four Principles with no subprinciples. It now contains 30 Rules as a replacement for the earlier Ethical Proscriptions. Matters of Ethical Propriety, separately specified in the earlier version, have been incorporated into the expressions of Principles and Rules. The 1992 rendition of this Code is a tighter, clearer, and a better public relations document than the earlier Code.

Basically the Code addresses professional responsibility to persons served, the general public, the profession, and espouses the intent to continued professional growth through education. It still, however, bears a strong paternalistic flavor and has elected for whatever reasons to ignore the modern trend expressed in codes of some other professions to allow for input from the consumer. Contrast it, for example, with the 1980 Code for Nurses of the American Nurses Association[2] reproduced in part as follows:

POINT 1

The nurse provides services with respect for human dignity and the uniqueness of the client unrestricted by considerations of social or economic status, personal attributes, or the nature of health problems.

> 1.1   Self-determination of Clients
> Whenever possible, clients should be fully involved in the overall planning and implementation of their own health care. Each client has the moral right to determine what will be done with his/her person; to be given the information necessary for making informed judgments; to be told the possible effects of care; and to accept, refuse, or terminate treatment. These same rights apply to minors and others not legally qualified and must be respected to the fullest degree permissible under law. The law in these areas may differ from state to state; each nurse has the obligation to be knowledgeable about and to protect and support the moral and legal rights of all clients under state laws and applicable federal laws, such as the 1974 Privacy Act. (p. 2)

The paragraph makes very clear that, although the nursing profession protects its professional role in health care delivery, there is respect and consideration for the rights of the client. The entire document is an excellent example of the current trend in the expression of professional ethics.

It is possible that such an expression of consumer empowerment is not a prudent consideration in some professions. The speech-language pathology and audiology professions may indeed be two of them. The 1992 ASHA Code of Ethics is not without other potential problems, however, exclusive of that consideration.

In Principle I, Rule B, for example, the advisability of using the word "ensure" could be questioned, as a practitioner's good-faith act of referring for a specific expertise can not *ensure*, that is, guarantee,

---

[2] American Nurses Association, Washington, DC.

high quality of service. Remember, one can fall below the high aspirations of a Principle, but failing to comply with a Rule may result in a violation, so it is best not to use potentially unachievable requisites in a Rule.

In Rule C it would appear that limiting professional service is justified as long as it is based on something other than the areas listed. In the same sense as saying too much can be the basis for problems, omissions also allow the growth of conduct that otherwise would not be condoned.

Principle II, Rule F, is perhaps less specific about calibration than it should be for a profession steeped in scientific accuracy. The statement is not good aesthetically, and it does very little to draw a distinction between the stringent requisites of audiology as a profession dealing, at least in part, with the measurement of auditory capacity and the sale of hearing aids as a business.

Principle III, Rule A is a clear departure from earlier versions, which indicated only academic degrees from accredited institutions would be recognized. The earlier position was an effort to rid the association of members whose degrees, particularly doctoral degrees, were achieved through nonstandard means, such as correspondence, academic credit awarded for years of experience, no residency fulfillment, and so forth. It is apparent from the Rule that the Association now believes instances of misrepresentation are better examined than qualifications of an academic institution.

Whether the footnote explanation of "misrepresentation" included in the Code will substitute effectively for the specificity lost in the revision of Principle III, Rule A remains to be seen. The footnote explanation of "misrepresentation" is, however, an excellent addition to the Code, regardless of the motivation for doing it.

Principle III, Rule B, probably needs more, not less, explanation, although there is reason to exercise caution over expressing too much. The area of conflict of interest is a difficult problem, and one that most practitioners who deal in product along with service find particularly irritating. The **appearance** of a conflict of interest is often as important as the act itself. The developers of the Code revision obviously felt that "proving" the appearance of a conflict of interest was too difficult, and opted to eliminate the phrase from the Code.

Overall the Code would read less monotonously and be more representative of the Association's values if the Principles were addressed to Members, rather than Individuals. The Principles should be values that the entire membership lives with. The Rules generally are meant to specify how the individual practitioner is expected to, or not to, behave in actual practice of the profession to support those Principles.

Although the points raised here may seem of limited consequence, the need for precise language and clearly stated expectations is important to the operation of the committee or board during deliberations for alleged noncompliance with the Code.

REPORTING PROCEDURES

The procedures generally followed by an ethics committee in carrying out its responsibilities are established to protect the rights of individuals brought before it for alleged ethics transgressions. Details on general internal processing of complaints is covered in a later chapter.

The procedures for reporting an alleged ethical violation are quite straightforward, however. Sometimes these procedures are part of the code, as is the case in the Code of Ethics of the AAA, and other times procedures for making an allegation are contained in a separate document.

Generally, all that is required in the initial reporting stages is to correspond with the committee, specifying the alleged violation and the person(s) involved—presenting as much factual information as available. Correspondence with the ethics committee is confidential.

The first step by the ethics committee in most procedures is a determination if the alleged misconduct involves the ethics code. If it does, it is then necessary to verify that the violation occurred as reported. This ideally entails obtaining documentation from several sources. The committee also needs to be presented with the alleged violator's side of the issue and will request an explanation from the person whose actions are being reported.

It is easy for committee members during deliberations of a particular case to become timid, that is, to become fearful of finding someone guilty of nonconformity to the Code, and to become reluctant to punish a violator, or to publish the finding and sanction of the committee. Conversely, sometimes a committee falls victim to one or two over-zealous committee members who think they should seek until they find a violation and then "throw the rascals out." Obvi-ously neither of these extremes should be tolerated, and fortunately the "seek-and-ye-shall-find" behavior is very infrequent.

Every committee also struggles with the moral and legal, as well as the ethical, issues surrounding cases. Additionally, a committee needs to determine the extent of their own involvement, that is, how far they should go in seeking information for settlement of an ethics transgression. These matters are discussed in the next chapter.

3

Ethical, Moral, and Legal Issues

The importance ascribed to illness expands, while the concept of fault shrinks.   (Lord Devlin)

Ethics committees should concern themselves with careful, firm ethics code enforcement because it is the right thing to do and because they have the right to do it. It is their responsibility to assure compliance with a code of ethics insofar as possible. To do so is in the best interests of all concerned.

In carrying out the duties of ethics code enforcement effectively and justifiably, however, committee members must keep in mind that their powers and even their roles are finite. There is very little that an ethics body can do to eradicate misconduct, but it can go a long way toward vindicating the values that result in rendering most people proud to be a member of a chosen profession. The task is difficult and most-members appointed to the responsibility of monitoring an association's ethics sometimes find the duties overwhelming. The job is made no less strenuous by the fact that some deviations from code compliance twist through not only ethical infractions, but moral and legal ones, and even malpractice as well.

Often the business of an ethics committee is made more difficult because those empowered with the job of ethics code enforcement fail to recognize that ethics committees do not provide the *only* forum for redressing disputes. The land is full of consumer agencies, courts, and other public arenas for resolving apparent wrongdoing. Ethics committees function best when employing resources to settle disputes involving professional ethics issues for which they have special expertise. In this capacity they provide the public's first line of defense, but certainly not the only one.

AN EXERCISE IN ETHICS

A brief exercise to engage in thinking about ethical conduct is often helpful. The following exercise has two purposes. First, it provides a change-of-pace from the material presented thus far, and second, it begins to establish a framework for later examples in this book, which deal with more complex ethical issues.

Read the following story carefully, remembering as much about the characters as you can. At the end of the story is a ranking to be completed and one or two questions for you to consider.

The Mousetrap

Once upon a time there was a handsome mouse named Drndl who lived with his wife and eight baby mice in the attic of a large mansion in the best part of town. Life was good for the family—not always fair, but good. Drndl foraged and provided for his family. The wife mouse, whose name was Marthalena, seemed happy. She stayed at home except for one day each week when she would leave the attic and be gone all day. She always returned with crumbs of bacon for the family.

On the morning of one day when Marthalena was supposed to be going out, Drndl said, "Marthalena, I must go to the church grounds today and look for my cousins. I will be gone all day until nightfall. You cannot go out today because I cannot be here to watch the babies. Do not leave the attic or I will be very angry when I return."

But Marthalena grew restless, and despite Drndl's warning, left the attic to visit, of all things, her lover in the basement of the nearby Country Club as she did one day of every week.

Her journey took her across the golf course, through a big patch of white sand, where she always left her tracks, past a flag sticking out of soft grass, which she regularly dug into because it felt good on her paws, and then on to a stream with a bridge. A man invariably stood at the end of the bridge and every week Marthalena had to scurry quickly to get past him and not be caught. Once safely over the bridge she had only then to run over a hill along a hard, black path, and into the hole between the stones under the window of what was called the Country Club.

Once inside, it was her habit to stop for a few minutes to speak with Madame Chardonnet, a Parisienne mouse she had met long ago on one of her many trips to the Club. Madame Chardie, as she was called by her mouse friends, lived in a little space apparently under the kitchen of the Country Club. Madame Chardie ran some sort of business. There were many male mice scurrying in and out all the time, and they all gave Madame Chardie money when they left.

It often smelled like bacon in the little space she occupied as living quarters, and there were always plenty of scraps around to eat. Madame Chardie was very generous with the bits of food, which likely fell from the kitchen above, and every week she gave Marthalena a small sack of bacon crumbs to take with her.

After a polite visit Marthalena left and continued down the dark passage to the place where her lover lived. She tapped on the door and when it opened she fell into the arms of Buckminster J. Ramigone, III, her lover. He kissed her on the muzzle, pushed the door closed with a flip of his hip, and pulled off her coat.

Several pleasant hours later Marthalena dressed and left. She scurried through the hole under the back window of the Club and ran as fast as she could over the hill and along the hard, black path to the bridge over the stream. But as she approached she could see that the man on the bridge now had a big shovel in his hands and he was blocking her path to the golf course.

"Aha, at last I'm going to get you," the man said. "No more running onto the greens for you! I'm going to fix you for good this time!"

He swung the shovel to the ground with great force. It just missed Marthalena who turned and ran all the way back to her lover for help.

"Our relationship is only a romantic one, my dear. And only once a week at that," Buckminster J. Ramigone, III said. "I will not risk my life. I cannot help!"

Marthalena frantically ran outside where she saw two mice rummaging through a trashcan. They looked up as she ran to them, panting.

"Help me help me," she pleaded. "I can't get over the bridge because there is a man there who will kill me with a big shovel if I go on the bridge to cross to the golf course. Come with me to the bridge and divert his attention so I can run across. I must get home! It's getting dark and I must be home!"

"We will do it," said the two grungy-looking mice, "but only if you will give us each $10."

"Ohhh, I do not have my purse with me. I have no money," Marthalena cried.

"That's too bad, Missie," said one of the mice. "We don't do nothin' for nothin'," said the other.

Marthalena fled back to Madame Chardonnet. She explained what was happening and asked her for $20 to pay for help from the two dirty mice.

Madame Chardonnet said, "Mon Dieu, ma petite, if you had not disobeyed your husband today, maybe none of this would have happened. It's your own fault, your own mess. I shall give you no money."

Marthalena was desperate. Night had fallen and the stars twinkled in the black sky above. She approached the bridge slowly. She saw no one there. Marthalena began to run as fast as she could to get across the bridge. Just as she bounced onto the bridge the man jumped from somewhere and slammed the shovel down on her little body and killed her.

Your task is to rate the behavior of the characters in the story from most ethical (1) to least ethical (6). It is an exercise to direct your thinking toward ethical behavior. Of course, there is no stated Code of Ethics here against which to compare the various behaviors, but from what you know so far about ethics go ahead and rank the behavior of the six characters below.

Drndl________   Marthalena________

Bridgeman________   Buckminster J. Ramigone, III________

Grungy mice________   Madame Chardonnet________

When you have ranked them to the best of your ability, consider whether the ranking changes if the prime consideration is moral, or legal behavior, rather than ethical. Do some behaviors equal others in rank when the reason for scaling shifts?[1] Is The Golden Rule sufficient to help with the ranking?

Chances are you ranked Drndl as the most ethical and Marthalena as the most unethical. That's a good start. Perhaps you felt the Bridgeman may have just been doing his duty to keep rodents off the greens. The lover, of course, is quite despicable, but is he unethical? Madame Chardie is a business lady, and the grungy mice are trying to make a dollar or two. There are moral, or immoral, explanations as well. Keep in mind that ethics is a system that attempts to control the behavior of a group according to principles on which members of the group have agreed.

TRANSGRESSIONS OF A DIFFERENT KIND

Having completed the exercise it should be easier to see that perhaps one of the most troublesome things for an ethics body to realize is that not every transgression by a professional is a professional trans-

---

[1] Don't look for an answer sheet. There isn't one. The whole book will help you find the answers, and they will be the best ones you are able to defend.

gression. Too frequently, for example, ethics committees are erroneously asked to deliberate such behavior as whether a member of a given professional association committed an unethical act because he or she sold a Jaguar with a defective transmission to a neighbor. In other words, there are some digressions from honorable conduct that are clearly not the business of an ethics committee. An ethics committee is obligated to know the difference.

Further, some professionals believe that if behavior is not illegal, then it certainly cannot be unethical. That belief is far removed from the fact. Stromberg (1990) indicates that, although certainly based on moral principles, the law itself is not a comprehensive moral code. Many legal behaviors, in fact, have been judged unethical.

Consider as an example an incident where a resident physician in urology at hospital A is taken to dinner along with residents from hospital B by a pharmaceutical representative from a company marketing a medication specific to diseases of the urinary bladder. Before dinner a slide and tape show of the efficacies of the drug is presented. The vice president for marketing of the drug company answers questions about the drug, praising its virtues in the treatment of even the most stubborn infections of the urinary tract.

Dinner is served, after which each resident is given a flower pot shaped like a human bladder and containing an amaryllis bulb. There is certainly nothing illegal in what the residents did. But is there a question of ethical impropriety? Perhaps, but many would choose to ignore it. There is also no malpractice or moral deviation. Why did the pharmaceutical representative take the residents to dinner; would it not have been as effective to have presented them with published data? Is the norm of reciprocity beginning to operate here?

As another example, nurses assigned to an operating room where large quantities of expendable supplies, medications, sterile items, and special instruments are used often find that lunch has been sent in to the area by one of the "detail reps" responsible for supplying many of the, let's say, suture packs. If the staff partakes of the lunch, is there an appearance of an ethics problem here? Probably. Is there an actual breach of ethics? Probably not, but there could be. Is the practice illegal? In no way.

Consider also these two examples. First, a Rand Corporation survey (Catlin, Bradbury, & Catlin, 1983) found that medical practitioners in HMOs with personal compensation packages encouraging them to avoid referring patients to specialists outside the system are **20% less** likely to detect depression and refer for specialized treatment than are fee-for-service physicians who do not have an antireferral incentive. Second, studies by the U.S. Department of Health and Human Services in 1984 and 1985 found that when doctors own clinical laboratories they order **45% more** lab tests for their patients than nonowners.

On the one hand, these behaviors are not illegal. On the other, they may be unethical. But there is also a chance that the conduct is just an indication of an economic reality, or a change in societal pressures.

There is the position, too, that folks who accept the lower health insurance cost of HMO coverage also accept that there will be some limitations to the extent of services they receive. But others would argue that low prices do not mean less-than-first-rate service. The practice of providing lower service is probably unethical, but there may be mitigating circumstances.

Just what is the ethical position in a situation such as this? Clearly, if patients are being denied care that is obviously necessary, and not specifically excluded from coverage by plan agreement, the ethical decision is straightforward. The matter becomes one of "quality of care," or as stated in some codes "the assurance that patients are referred for care beyond the practitioner's expertise." ASHA's Code and the Code of the AAA have similar wording. Most ethics committees would agree that low charge for service does not in and of itself justify a breach of ethics.

Judgments are not often that matter-of-fact, however. In areas involving cost-benefit trade-offs the waters become murky in considering ethical, legal, and even moral considerations. For instance, what happens when an HMO hires an otologic surgeon who has great expertise in head and neck surgery, but not in surgical techniques involving the ear? Is it not the ethical course for the patient requiring ear surgery to be referred to the "best" otologic surgeon in town? But how can an ethics committee find a practitioner in violation of an ethics stipulation when the practice procedure is the policy of an employer?

There have already been several litigations alleging that health care providers are liable for setting up a system that by virtue of its procedures leads to denial of needed care. In other words, it is the employer, not the practitioner, who is at fault. The decisions of the courts are varied on the issue, and, in any case, an organization's code only has authority over its members.

The ethics question that permeates the issue is, of course, whether the consumers in this situation are fully aware that they are not always getting what they think they are getting. After all, ethics codes have as one of their primary duties the protection of the public.

Many times an appealing compromise is simply to require that practitioners provide full disclosure of the economic constraints that might bear on patient treatment, or the ethics of practice. That is a question that each ethics committee must answer for itself, however—taking into account the stresses of the times and the degree of public dependence on them for protection, as well as the implications such a requirement might impose on professional job security. The hard course quite clearly is to hold all professionals, regardless of economic context or legal finding, to fundamental norms of the profession.

One of the reasons this is easier said than done is that much of the effort by professional associations is befuddled by the wispy relationship of the law, licensure stipulations, jurisdictional regulatory bodies, malpractice, morals, and ethics. A professional alleged to have violated a code of ethics may attempt to evade the process by protesting that a charge cannot be made because the individual was acquitted in a court proceeding for the same alleged offense. Or a complainant may ask an ethics committee to *get* someone for unethical conduct because the person isn't licensed. An ethics committee member may believe that a citation of unethical behavior is a foregone conclusion in a specific case found guilty of malpractice by a jury of the court. It probably would be, but it doesn't *have* to be. These positions are additionally confused by the multiple intersecting realms in which problems of professional misconduct can be addressed.

ETHICAL, MORAL, AND LEGAL OVERLAP

Figure 3–1 displays the relationship among illegal, unethical, and malpractice transgressions. Obviously, a practice behavior can be any one of these, to the exclusion of the others; any two of them to the exclusion of the third; or, all three as represented by the overlapping areas of the squares.

A conduct may be tacky, or even repugnant, but not be actionable under civil law. Wearing shorts and a tank top to the office might be an example. Another conduct may be professionally unethical or even malpractice and neutral to the requirements of a licensing law. Such things as a professional knowingly holding membership in a discriminatory club, or the fraudulent sale of a personal item would be examples of behaviors falling into this category. Incidents might also include professional conduct such as continually belittling other practitioners. Such examples, however, are not to indicate that **all** nonadmirable behavior is exempt from moral or legal rules.

Some conduct clearly outside the ethical rules of an association, as well as the licensing laws, malpractice standards, and even criminal law, however, may be civilly actionable; that is, it confers on the injured party the right to sue for suitable remedy. Examples of this

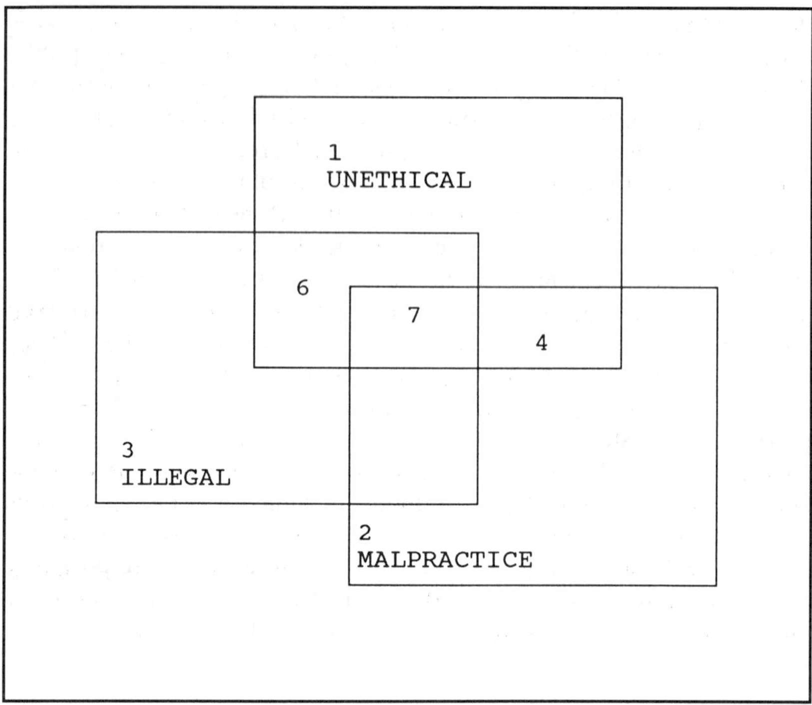

Figure 3–1. Diagrammatic presentation of the relationship among sanctioned conducts. Behavior can be either unethical (1) malpractice (2) or illegal (3). Area overlap indicates conduct can also be unethical and malpractice (4) malpractice and illegal (5) illegal and unethical (6) or all three (7) unethical, illegal and malpractice.

type of conduct would be a breach of an HMO employment contract, for instance, or failure to deliver a finished oil painting to a gallery despite receiving an advance payment. Some instances of civilly actionable conduct also breach moral and ethical standards as well; fraudulent billing, would be an example.

Conduct that is primarily personal and not professional may be unlawful but not unethical, not malpractice, and not contrary to the stipulations required to maintain a license to practice. Violating a court order concerning alimony payment, child support, or disturbing the peace are examples. Conduct may be unlawful, but not in the sense of "criminally unlawful," and would not trigger an ethical action. Failure to file an income tax might fall into this category. Driving while intoxicated might, however, invoke an ethical citation from a professional association, as might a traffic citation, depending on the strength and conviction of the association.

It might be considered unethical in some arenas to take on so many patients in a practice that the total quality management of patients suffers. Such conduct would not, in most instances, be judged malpractice, morally wrong, or contrary to most licensing statutes.

Deceptive advertising may not be illegal, or even amoral or malpractice. It is quite probably unethical, and may, in addition, violate some state licensing laws.

Some states having licensing jurisdiction over professions require practitioners to file periodic reports with the state. Failure to do so is an obvious violation of the licensing law. It would be reaching for the extreme, however, for an ethics committee to find that conduct unethical.

Some behavior might be unethical and malpractice but not violate the law. There are harmless technical ethics violations, such as the failure of a Clinical Fellowship Year (CFY) supervisor (in the case of the American Speech-Language-Hearing Association) to perform according to the reasonable expectations of the fellow, which is not generally actionable from a legal standpoint, but may be found by an ethics committee to be unethical. Also there are mistaken or biased jury verdicts in malpractice cases, which should not automatically incite licensure sanctions or ethics citations.

Conduct may be unethical, illegal, malpractice, and immoral. Having sexual relations with patients would certainly qualify in this category.

Failure of an otherwise meticulous researcher to provide information necessary for informed consent might be considered as an episode of malpractice or a violation of a licensing statute, but not be unethical in the broadest sense. On the other hand, some ethics codes clearly stipulate that members shall provide the information necessary to enable consumers to make informed choices. Failure to do so by the practitioner would result in an ethics committee's finding of noncompliance with the code. Such conduct could conceivably result in a jury finding of negligence also—if the case went that far.

It should be clear that the interweaving of ethical, moral, and legal concerns constantly accompanies the deliberations of ethics committees. The recurring question is always which process is the most appropriate for the redress of cases involving professional misconduct. Stated another way, ethics committees have the right to judge an alleged violation to be outside their jurisdiction.

ISSUES OF DEFENSE

The matters of ethical, moral, and legal overlap are certainly key to the issue of an ethics committee's decision of when and where to begin and stop. Even though these committees represent the public's first line of defense, that responsibility carries with it an obligation for ethics committees to be aware of the many ramifications of their actions or, for another matter, their inactions.

Should, for example, an ethics committee process an alleged violation of professional ethics in a case that has been delayed for years in the courts? In other words, is "timeliness" considered as an effective deterrent to ethics prosecution? Lawyers will affirm that a professional misconduct case may remain active for years before a verdict is reached (Stromberg, 1990).

Timeliness

It is conceivable, in hypothetical example, for Dr. Green to commit an act of misconduct in 1983, for a complaint by a patient who alleges Green guilty of alcohol abuse on the job to be filed with the state licensing board in 1985, for a hearing to be held in 1986, and an order against Green to be issued by the licensing board in 1987. Dr. Green then initiates a lawsuit alleging "procedural error," and a court sets aside the licensing board order in 1988. A settlement is reached in 1989 in which Dr. Green admits misconduct, admits to being in treatment, and swears to have been free from substance abuse since the incident. The professional association learns of the matter in 1989 and brings action through their ethics committee in 1990. Dr. Green, although admitting guilt of misconduct to the ethics committee, pleads for the association not to force a repeat of the whole thing again—especially since the misconduct transpired seven years ago.

Legal advisors to ethics committees generally would agree that, unless the delay violates the procedures of the committee for filing complaints, lapse of time should not be substantive grounds to remove the jurisdiction of an ethics committee. The real question revolves around whether it makes sense to penalize an individual further for misconduct in 1983, if the cause of the misconduct has been removed since at least 1987. In general, the passage of time is not always reason enough to prevent action by an ethics committee. Compassion may be yet another matter.

Illness

There is still another concern that ethics committees must be aware of in their sensitivity to the boundaries of ethical, legal, and moral issues. This is that the concept of illness seems to be expanding at the same rate at which the concept of moral fault is shrinking. What the hypothetical Dr. Green is also saying in the plea is that the sickness (impairment) was so compelling the wrong was not recognized, but when Dr. Green did realize it (because of being caught), the offender stopped the wrongful act and enrolled in a treatment program. Therefore, Dr. Green believes there was nothing unethical. The individual is not at fault because of sickness.

To a degree professional ethics committees should show empathy toward members afflicted with physical or mental health problems, but in most cases affliction does not excuse the bad conduct. Members of professional associations, especially those in health care fields, have a moral obligation to self-awareness. Personal problems must be recognized and solved before resulting in harm to the very persons who seek professional help. Failure of a professional to recognize the existence of a personal trait or habit deterring provision of quality care should not be sufficient to repel ethics committee intervention.

SCOPE OF PRACTICE

The scope of practice of a particular profession provides another area which crosses ethical, legal, and moral boundaries. Most professionals are eager to expand their scope of practice, while most ethics committees deem it their duty to prevent professionals from expanding beyond their training and expertise. The dilemma is real because a profession's scope of practice is made up not only of what it is competent by training to do, but what the state law **allows** it to do. Often academia leads in creating the problem by teaching new procedures to those still in training. Legislative mandate lags behind, making it possible for a practitioner to be held in violation of the law, but not in noncompliance with an ethics code that might allow them to do anything for which they have been properly trained.

Sometimes ethics committees become the battleground for turf wars between professions. Stromberg (1990) gives three examples:

1. Optometrists and ophthalmologists have fought over whether optometrists can prescribe eye-related drugs. (*American Optometric Association v. FTC*, 1980)
2. In Michigan physiatrists and physical therapists (PTs) have litigated over whether PTs can perform electromyography. (*Palazzo v. Teasdale*, 1989)
3. California psychologists and psychiatrists have litigated over whether psychologists should have staff privileges and be able to treat their patients independently in hospitals. (*California Association of Psychology Providers v. Rank*, 1990)

As tempting as it may be for ethics committees to become involved in handing out sanctions against those who step beyond the scope of accepted practice, such battles are better joined in courtroom and legislative arenas. Ethics committees need to be clear that their function is to enforce existing legal and ethical limits, not to expand or contract the scope of practice.

ADVERTISING

Advertising is said to be among the top areas for complaints to ethics committees. In general, however, it is not the poor image created by the advertisement that motivates the complaint. In many instances it is other mistreatment the patient has undergone causing the complainant to contact the ethics committee. An unrealized benefit described in the practitioner's ad is then thrown in. But it is often of secondary importance.

Advertising and marketing are becoming common to professional practice, unlike the situation 25 years ago. Today at least 13% of attorneys, 11% of physicians, 23% of dentists, and 34% of optometrists advertise and conduct some type of marketing process. Virtually all audiologists and speech-language pathologists who operate a private practice as the sole means of support advertise or undertake other marketing strategies.

The most effective media as judged by professionals who advertise are the yellow pages (37%), newspapers, including shoppers' guides (19%), direct mail (15%), and TV (9%). In a 1985 survey by *McChesney* magazine, 96% of readers favored advertising by professionals on the grounds that it provided them with useful information on which to base a choice of where to go for what.

Professionals have a right to advertise. This right is given to them by the Constitution. Private organizations cannot unreasonably restrain trade, but they can police advertising to eliminate what is false, deceptive, or misleading. The Federal Trade Commission (FTC) in its 1980 suit (American Medical Association, 1980) against the AMA for restricting the freedom of doctors to advertise ultimately agreed that the association could engage in:

> ...formulating, adopting, disseminating to its constituent and component medical organizations and to its members, and enforcing reasonable ethical guidelines governing...[that which the AMA...reasonably believes would] be false or deceptive...to actual or potential patients, who, because of their particular circumstance are vulnerable to undue influence. (p. 96)

Ethically and legally in most sectors, an ad is unlawful if it is deceptive, false, or misleading. It is probably morally wrong as well to advertise that something is what it isn't. The FTC (1984) has declared that it will regard a statement as deceptive if there is misrepresentation, omission, or other practice that is likely to mislead the consumer. Recall that the Code of Ethics of the ASHA (1992) contains a footnote defining "misrepresentation" in much these same terms.

But an ad is not deceptive simply because some consumer misinterprets it, or merely because some people, because of ignorance or incomprehension, may be misled by an honest claim. As the FTC (1984) has pointed out, perhaps a few misguided souls believe all Danish Pastry is made in Denmark, but that is not sufficient justification for a claim of false advertising.

Increasingly, professional associations and professionals themselves try to stimulate indirect advertising by cultivating opportunities for interviews and other forms of public forum, which provide an indirect means to speak of their practices. Ethics committees are sometimes asked to slap the hands of practitioners who make claims during media interviews that are clearly misleading. When cited, respondents will usually claim the statement was inadvertent and prompted by the nervousness of the moment. Repeated misleading statements, however, call for the ethics committee to make a cautionary statement to the individual.

From another viewpoint, ethical, moral, and legal concerns may face the professional employed in large bureaucratic institutions such as industrial corporations, universities, or government agencies. These environments may include situations that could involve a possible law violation. Public disclosure of information relating to professional staff may be damaging to the employer, for example. Although a legal settlement might include a gag order on all publicity related to a particular incident, there is still the matter of ethics to confront with the practitioner's association. Examples of this situation might include some internal impropriety or manufacture, advertisement, and distribution of a device with a known design flaw, discovered when someone has blown the whistle.

The professional caught in such a situation is similar to a worm on a hot rock. No matter what position is assumed, it's still hot. It also may incite an ethics infraction.

Summary

In summary, professionals set forth criteria in their code of conduct that often determine the decision-making process. Professions assure conformity with a codified set of rules by specifying sanctions for persons who make decisions that jeopardize the public. Uniformity of expectations is focused by support for legal or licensing status, or by some other credential, such as admission to the profession. This is evidenced by examination, registration, and graduation from an accredited curriculum, according to an article written by R. H. McCuen (1983).

In a purely technical sense, all professionals are educated to solve problems. The motivation to do so derives from a commitment to serve and an obligation to maintain professional integrity in all situations involving co-workers, employers, those served, and ultimately society, itself. Thus it is critical that professionals maintain a sensitivity to the need for strong moral, ethical, and legal judgment. To do so easily translates into principled professional conduct.

MAKING THE FINDINGS KNOWN

It is necessary to understand a few points concerning the moral, legal, and ethical obligations a committee has toward making its findings known in a particular case. It is not unusual for ethics committees to be timid publicly stating their decisions. Committees become wary of potential litigation or threats of law suits that might be mounted by respondents, and can slow nearly to a halt when the moment arrives to make their sanctions public.

In general, the attitude is not worthy of a group entrusted with monitoring the conduct of a profession. In cases of peer review concerning certain types of misconduct by physicians, in fact, reporting to a federal Disciplinary Data Bank is now mandated by the Health Care Quality Improvement Act. Nonphysician health care groups in 1992 still enjoy the option of reporting disciplinary actions involving practitioners.

In one respect failure to report seems to flaunt one of the prime rationales for a code of ethics. If the committee is shy about making its decisions public, it may also be shy about making decisions. It is, after all, a public service to inform colleagues that a practitioner to whom they may make referrals has been judged guilty of ethics misconduct. In the case of *Kreuzer v. The American Academy of Periodontology* (1984) the court said:

> This court will not infer a conspiracy to violate antitrust laws based on a showing of contact between two independent professional associations on matters of mutual interests and concern. This is the very purpose and nature of professional associations and this court will erect no barriers to accomplishment of this. (p. 1489)

The finding of the court set a valuable precedent for the exchange of information among organizations having similar professional interests and aims.

Professional ethics committees have a qualified privilege to communicate the results of their deliberations. Needless disclosures, however, may very well form the basis for litigious action from the respondent. The rule of thumb is to communicate carefully and consistently in accordance with pre-established procedures.

The need for professional ethics, the need to communicate about the conduct of professionals, and the need for professionals to know more about the ethics of their profession should be apparent. The knowledge and specialized skills required to practice a profession are clearly reflected in professional curricula, internship programs, continuing education requirements, and scientific workshops held by most professions to instill the state-of-the-art in its practitioners. At the same time, the professions have been slow to acknowledge the value of the decisions they make in the practice of their chosen fields.

Graduate education programs include few formal courses in the most critical area of professional ethics. The need for professionals to understand and appreciate the ethical, moral, and legal strategies that apply in selecting a path to ethically correct and professionally acceptable decisions seems to be a much needed area for development in the professional arena.

4

Jurisdiction, Diversity, and Some Other Ethics Concerns

Unite tenderness with steadiness, and condescension with authority. (Thomas Percival)

The Ethical Practice Board of a professional organization has an obligation to inform the membership on issues that shape the functioning of the board as well as areas bearing on the implementation of a code of professional behavior. The membership has the right to know as much as possible about the matters of professional ethics that concern an Ethical Practice Board or committee. Among those matters, the areas of **jurisdiction** of power and **diversity** of practice are important for the understanding of professional ethics.

Many ethicists devote considerable discussion to the topic of jurisdiction as it applies to the authority of an ethics body in looking beyond the strict boundaries of a particular profession. A similar intensity of discussion is not afforded to the topic of diversity, however. Carl Stromberg (1990) sheds considerable light on both subjects as both relate to the practice of a profession. That relationship will be explored and extended in this chapter.

JURISDICTION

In the matter of jurisdiction ethics monitors are concerned with the question, "How far into the lives of professional practitioners should an Ethical Practice Board be allowed to go?" Professional practitioners do not like anyone looking over their shoulder in professional life. Surely the objection is magnified when extended beyond the profession and into private life. Similarly, no member of an Ethical Practice Board should ever need to assume the role of a proactive monitor of the everyday life of a professional.

In some professions there seems to be wariness of Ethical Practice Board members by the general membership. The membership often sees the board as a cloak-and-dagger group shrouded in mystery, lurking in the shadows, and capable of ending a professional career with the stroke of a pen. This is an unfortunate interpretation and should never be the image fostered by an Ethical Practice Board.

First of all, it is a false image. No board acts in this manner. There are sufficient checks and balances built into the system of ethics monitoring to guard against careless or unjustified decisions and sanctions. Although much of the work of a board on a particular alleged violation of a code is confidential, confidentiality is maintained for the protection of the individuals involved, not merely to maintain an atmosphere of secrecy. Confidentiality has nothing to do with hiding the activities of the board from the membership for any reason other than a respondent's right to privacy.

Second, most, but not all, professional organizations allow for an appeal process for ethics code violations. The appeal process provides for a reconsideration of the facts, if there has been an error in the process. In essence it is an escape valve to allow for correction of processing errors or errors in severity of sanction. Boards must always be able to justify their findings. They do not and cannot operate independently or in a showy fashion that permeates society in an effort to seek, find, and punish members of a professional group (Stromberg, 1988; Wright, 1987).

Practitioners, if given a choice, probably would opt for an arrangement where ethics monitors have no jurisdiction outside the workplace. Unfortunately, the attitude, "What I do on my own time is my own business," understates the value of a Code of Ethics. It is a simplification to support the position that anything happening outside the workplace is beyond the concern and jurisdiction of professional ethics. The viewpoint that *nothing* beyond the workplace is material for an ethics committee to consider may be still prevalent, but it is far too narrow to be beneficial in today's society.

One needs only to consider the possible consequences in a few hypothetical examples of off-duty behavior to realize that on-the-job performance could easily be influenced. Even though the behavior in the following examples would probably take place away from the work environment, the risk of an ethics infraction would be quite high by the standards embodied in most codes. Consider:

> An active cardiac transplant surgeon who becomes regularly involved in weekend substance abuse.

> A speech-language pathologist who treats children in a private practice is known to be a child abuser.

> A civil engineer who designs public highways is found guilty of loan sharking.

> An audiologist who sells hearing aids in the office of a physician is under investigation for participation in child pornography.

These behaviors might be relevant to the performance of the individual's professional duties even though the activities in question would occur outside the work environment. The position that what one does on one's own time is not the business of an ethics board seems an inappropriate stance, if the public is, indeed, to be protected.

At the opposite extreme of the jurisdiction question, that is, if *everything* outside the workplace is to be the fair concern of an Ethical Practice Board, it is possible to state a broader standard. For example, "All conduct implicates professional ethics if it affects the workplace, even if it occurred outside the job environment." *That* view may be a good one. However, it requires the Ethical Practice Board of an association to *prove* that an outside conduct actually resulted in, or was the cause of, harm to the recipient of the professional services in a given case. The point is that proof must be found tying the misconduct to an episode of harmful service (Fletcher, 1966).

In the hypothetical case of the substance-abusing cardiac surgeon, for instance, the board would be required to first prove that harm was done to the person by the surgeon, and second that the surgeon harmed the patient *because* of the substance abuse that occurred off duty. Similar logic and the need for cause-and-effect proof can be applied to the other cases as well.

This is not an easy task for an Ethical Practice Board. Proof obviously depends heavily on information obtained from expert sources. Once a connection is proven, however, jurisdiction is not in doubt. Clearly the best interest of the patient would not be uppermost in the practitioner's mind in the above examples, if proven. It is likely that the ethics of the professional association would be citable in each of the examples.

Another difficult problem arises when there is a known bad private conduct that has not *yet* caused harm, but may do so in the future. In other words, if there is sufficient knowledge among the colleagues of the speech-language pathologist in the example that several incidents of child abuse have occurred outside the workplace, is it the responsibility of those colleagues to report a possible ethics violation in an effort to *prevent* one that is likely to transpire?

The potential risks to the colleagues are obvious, but they may be no greater than the potential risks to the consumer of services. One must also speculate what might happen if the situation is brought to light for other reasons by other persons, and it is **then** discovered that the colleagues knew about the matter for some time. Their failure to report the problem may put them at risk of violating the code also.

Clearly, Ethical Practice Boards as well as practitioners, are faced with difficult choices. If nothing beyond the work setting is justifiably the concern of the Ethical Practice Board, there is great potential risk that the Code of Ethics will have a limited effect on enhancing the image of the profession.

At the opposite end of the continuum, if everything outside the practice environment is to be considered the concern of an ethics board a great deal of information must be amassed by the board, in every reported ethical violation. They just won't be able to collect needed information because of financial constraints, the right to privacy, and general reluctance of monitoring bodies to share information. Moreover, limits that committees and boards place on themselves by their voluntary status are difficult to surmount.

The "everything is fair game so watch out" view is burdensome to the boards. It is too all-encompassing to support morally, legally, or ethically. There still exist some codes with an even more liberal position, however. Although found in older versions of ethics codes, the position is to sanction for "any conduct that demeans the profession in the view of the public." It's a variation of the "everything" approach, but with the added variable that the *public* all but brands the practitioner merely by reporting a misconduct.

Fortunately modern boards recognize that a statement such as the above is too vague to be an enforceable standard. Vague, subjective standards are gradually being phased out of the codes of most professions and replaced by objective statements of accepted behavior and prohibitions against those behaviors deemed unacceptable to the practice.

The Jurisdiction Guidepost

The most defensible position on the question of jurisdiction is that an ethics board should be empowered to consider *any* conduct by a professional member of an organization—wherever it occurs—if the behavior:

A. Impairs professional functioning, or
B. Betrays the stated values that the profession is on record to uphold.

As a general rule, ethics codes and the individuals responsible for monitoring professional conduct view these two points as guidelines in the process of deciding questions of jurisdiction.

DIVERSITY

Another issue to be considered by ethics boards is the area of **diversity** within a profession. This matter concerns how much a code of ethics should accommodate the variety of a profession. Frequently, practicing individuals argue that ethics committees, in general, do not fully appreciate the special circumstances of a particular practicing group or of specific geographic locales.

In other words, there is a feeling among some practitioners that the circumstances of a practice should mitigate or even eliminate certain ethical conformities within that practice when the circumstances are shown to be beyond the control of the practitioner. Additionally, some feel that the special circumstances of a specific practice offer an even better level of care for the consumer of service than would be the case if ethics conformities were applied.

A test case in point might be that an Ethical Practice Board would have to judge whether it is acceptable for a podiatrist, for instance, to prescribe corrective shoes and also profit from dispensing the product if practicing in rural North Dakota, where the only alternative for a patient in need of specially fabricated prescriptive shoes is a shoe store 300 miles away. Assuming that the sale of product is prohibited by the ethics code governing the practice of podiatry, the practitioner could plead that: (1) It is better for the consumer to buy the shoes in the office than to drive 300 miles to have the prescription satisfied by an orthopedic shoe store, or (2) That the geographic location of the practice is such that a deviation from the ethics rule should be allowed.

The issue is clearly whether it is ethical for the person who prescribes the special shoes, in this case the podiatrist, and the person who sells the shoes, also in this case the podiatrist, to benefit in a material way from both circumstances. In other words, is there an element of conflict of interest raised by selling the shoes prescribed, and if there is, can it be overlooked from the ethical viewpoint because the circumstances are unique?

The board would need to judge the credibility of the argument and basically determine whether allowing the practice to continue would set a precedent. In the event a second podiatrist opened an office in the same or even a nearby town, the board would be powerless to prevent that office from selling shoes also, if it had allowed the first one to do it in the name of a special need. Maybe that would be justified. Perhaps it wouldn't.

Other things also would need to be considered by an ethics committee in this case. There would be the question of whether the "special need" is still present for the second podiatrist, as the first podiatrist could sell shoes for both practices.

The board also would need to determine whether there would be potential infringement on development and growth in the commercial sector by condoning the sale of prescription shoes in the podiatry practice. Questions concerning the possible legal entanglements faced by the ethics committee in this situation, and the implications for violation of antitrust laws need answers. Obviously the committee would require legal advice before proceeding. That requirement is yet another constraint ethics boards must face. Legal advice is expensive, often slow in reaching a conclusion, and many times necessitates the collection of more information than the committee is able to acquire easily.

From a philosophical point of view, the board would need to consider whether the practice of a podiatrist selling shoes is defendable from an ethical position in North Dakota, but not in New York City, Baltimore, or Nashville, for example.

Another case in point concerning the diversity issue might involve the audiologist in a rural school district who during routine hearing screening asks that each child repeat, "Theophilus Thistle, the thistle sifter, thrust three thousand thistles through the thick of his thumb." Based on the quality of the recitation the audiologist labels the child as "speech defective," and requests a medical consultation. The rationale posed by the audiologist is that professional duties are performed in a remote section of the United States and if the audiologist didn't make these judgments, no one would.

Reliance on the uniqueness of a practice becomes a crucial matter, but the board can never be so sensitive to the diversity imposed by people, places, and things that it judges everything to be an ethically acceptable behavior just because there is some narrow reason to support it. On the other hand, categorical dismissal of a unique procedure for the sole reason that it doesn't conform to the mainstream is a mistake of equal magnitude.

OTHER CONCERNS

A situation often confronting the Ethical Practices Board of the American Speech-Language-Hearing Association is whether a certified speech-language pathologist can ethically test for hearing threshold by air and bone conduction in a rural school population and descriptively report the results simply because there is no audiologist available to the community for several hundred miles. The rationale usually provided is that children in the small rural school district simply would not have a hearing test unless the speech-language pathologist conducts it. Speech-language pathologists who function in this manner feel they are qualified to provide the service, because they, at least, have *some* training, and they are only "screening."

That, too, becomes a point of question as bone conduction testing and reporting of results other than pass/fail also may be involved. The association's Code of Ethics clearly indicates that it is unethical for practitioners to provide services in areas for which they do not hold the Certificate of Clinical Competence. There can be, however, extenuating circumstances, such as utilizing the consultative services of an audiologist to oversee the hearing screening activity.

To the Ethical Practice Board of the American Speech-Language-Hearing Association, this type of apparent violation of the Code is known as "crossover." The term defines instances in which members provide service in a field for which they do not hold the Certificate of Clinical Competence. Crossover represents the most frequent ethics violation cited among that association's speech-language pathologists and audiologists.

There is no aspect of the speech-language pathology or audiology fields that is untouched by some aspect of the Code of Ethics of either the ASHA, or the AAA. The areas of diagnosis, testing, management of patients/clients, administration, research, supervision, publication, and so forth, are all addressed to some degree, and it is in the best interests of practitioners to be familiar with the stipulations of their Code of Ethics. Ignorance of the code, or the "Gee, I didn't know I couldn't do that" attitude after one has been cited for a violation is not a valid defense in any profession.

Another area of the ASHA code that receives a high activity level sometimes related to the diversity of the practice is the area of Clinical Fellowship Year (CFY) supervision. More frequently than one might expect, the ASHA ethics group receives a letter from members in a CFY who complain that their supervisor refused to sign the CFY form following completion of the experience, and "no reason was given." The distraught CFY, of course, claims that the conduct is unprofessional, uncalled for, and unethical. Most of the time the CFY is correct, the behavior is unethical, if, in fact, no reason was given and the disapproval came as a surprise to the fellow.

Efforts of the ethics committee to obtain an explanation from the CFY supervisor often reaps little more than a description of the uniqueness of the particular setting, that is, the diversity in the practice. The supervisor was "too busy" because the practice "suddenly took on a new contract." Rarely is there a plausible excuse to make ethical something that is clearly unethical. There is little defense for allowing a CFY person to function for the entire year and at the end of the experience inform the fellow that the CFY experience cannot be approved because of poor performance during the year.

Some audiology and speech-language practitioners spend a great deal of time on the road traveling from one nursing home, extended care facility, or hospital to another. Some, in order to cover as many facilities as possible in one day, virtually leave the motor running in their vehicle, hurry into the nursing home, look at a patient and run out. At the end of the week or month, the billing notices are turned in. Occasionally fraudulent billing occurs—billing for service not rendered.

A respondent cited for fraudulent billing tries to take refuge in the diversity of the practice. Some practitioners believe their practice is too busy to conform to ethics rules. Others feel they spend so much time in travel that they can't get their records completed when they see the patient and don't finish the notes until a month later. In other words, every practitioner believes a uniqueness exists in their practice that will provide the mitigating circumstance to support a deviation from the ethics of their profession.

At least once, ethics monitors have deliberated a case of fraudulent billing in which the practitioner billed a nursing home patient for a "cognitive retraining" session that, according to the record, took place two days after the patient had expired. Medicare refused to reimburse the nursing home. The home billed the patient's next of kin who looked at the dates of billed services and contacted the Ethical Practices Board.

Practices are reported in which full fees are charged for services provided by students who are not directly supervised, unnecessary services are provided to terminal patients, misrepresented services are provided, and so on. In most instances the cited practitioner explains that his or her practice is set up with the cited procedure as the only means to meet the needs of the community or to accomplish the task. Seldom does that prove to be the actual situation.

In most fields there are widely diverse professional approaches to service, and lively debates are mounted regularly on the most effective methods. In a few instances ethics codes have settled the issues.

However, ethics codes should not be used as a mechanism to stifle healthy diversity, or to prevent practice adjustments necessary to meet modern needs by penalizing professional behavior that is not absolutely mainstream. Neither, however, should Ethical Practice Boards be intimidated by a cry for pluralism.

In some professional fields that have by tradition maintained a close business relationship with product suppliers and manufacturers, the issues surrounding the business and professional aspects of a practice fall into the category of diversity, at least to a degree.

Audiologists, for example, who by ethics code restrictions prior to 1991 were not allowed to dispense hearing aids, now through revision of the code, are supported in the selling of products they prescribe. The revision was not won by waving a banner for diversity, but rather by recognizing that the practice of audiology in providing service to the hearing impaired population required the dispensing of hearing aids despite code prohibitions.

As other nonmedical services to the hearing impaired are provided by audiologists, it seems a logical extension that they be allowed by ethics code to dispense hearing aids as well. Today they are allowed to sell the product. In several states they also must be licensed as commercial vendors, a somewhat degrading requirement.

An interesting point in this regard is the obvious fact that some audiologists were actually cited many years ago by the Ethical Practices Board of the American-Speech-Language-Hearing Association for dispensing hearing aids, which in those days was a clear violation of the Code of Ethics (Curran & Harford, 1991). Today those same audiologists would be in compliance with the code because the sale of hearing aids by audiologists is no longer prohibited.

The question posed by nonprofessionals was if the practitioners were truly acting unethically during the time they were dispensing hearing aids. As the code was changed some years later to allow for dispensing of products, the assumption is that professionals must have been doing the right thing. The supposition is off the mark.

The situation is similar to being cited for exceeding the 55 mph speed limit and paying a fine. If the speed limit is increased to 65 mph a year later, were you obeying the law when you were cited at 55 mph? The answers are obvious in the case of the speeding violation and the ethical violation involving audiologists dispensing hearing aids at a time in the audiology field when that practice was not ethical.

By accepting licensure and certification within a profession, a practitioner also accepts the commitment to uphold the value and scope of practice of that profession, so indicates Wright (1987). The value statements and the scope of practice of a profession are meant to protect the public and to ensure insofar as possible that the public does not think it is getting something more than is actually provided. An Ethical Practice Board expects that practitioners function within the stipulations of a current code.

DIVERSITY SCENARIOS

Those who operate as private practitioners are more likely to experience ethics citations. This is because competition among practitioners is greater, as are the temptations, and because the private practitioner is more visible. Additionally, the checks and balances of professional practices in institutions such as hospitals, university programs, and local and federal governments are generally, but not always, more encompassing than those in private practice. The military and the Veterans' Administration have the most stringent on-the-job rules and therefore rarely, if ever, are practitioners in these environments found in noncompliance with the code of ethics.

Examples of diversity to consider in the following almost true cases:

Case 1: The Summer Program

Fictional "Mrs. Trudy Smith," a certified speech-language pathologist from Montana treated a pool of 45 children in a Montana school district during the academic year. The district Department of Education had no summer program, so the children received no treatment. But shrewd "Mrs. Smith" maintained a private practice during the summer months and offered to treat the children for a fee. Most of them accepted.

The next school year the census of children needing attention by the speech therapist rose to 97. The school hired fictional "Mrs. Brown" to assist "Mrs. Smith" during the year.

That summer, because of the number of children in need of speech services, the Department of Education continued the speech program for the children during the vacation. The summer school program was run by "Mrs. Brown." "Mrs. Smith" also maintained her private practice. Thirty-five children were treated by her in private therapy rather than at the school's free therapy program.

Fictional "Mrs.Brown" reported fictional "Mrs. Smith" to the Ethical Board of the Association saying she was unprofessional for taking patients away from school for her own personal financial gain. Was "Mrs. Smith" guilty of an ethics infraction?[1]

---

[1] No. Parents of children were given a choice of either the school program for free, or Smith's for a fee. Thirty-five of them chose to pay. There is no ethics violation here.

Case 2: To Be or Not To Be?

"Ginger Johnson" is a CFY about to finish and open a private practice. A final conference is scheduled with her CFY supervisor, but "Ginger," for reasons not relevant, missed the conference. Her supervisor will not sign the completed CFY form as approved because "Ginger" missed the final conference.

To make matters worse, the new Yellow Pages of the telephone directory have been published, and "Ginger" is listed as: "Ginger Johnson, MS, CCC-A. Audiologist." "Mr. Rogers," an adjunct professor at the university, sees the listing and blows the whistle on "Ginger." "Rogers" claims "Johnson" is violating the code section dealing with misrepresentation, deception, fraud, and so forth. "Johnson" says she didn't want to miss the opportunity for an ad in the telephone book so she had sent the information in a long time ago knowing she would be finished sometime. What do you think? Who is unethical?[2]

Case 3: When Is Fitting not Fitting?

"Barney Smith," an audiologist in a hospital program, fits a programmable hearing aid to a 47-year-old man whose services are being paid for by contract arrangement that the audiologist holds with an HMO. The contract was negotiated for a fixed charge for services, and the invoice cost of hearing aids plus an agreed overhead mark-up, but not to exceed a certain dollar amount. In addition, "Barney" agreed not to charge the HMO subscriber the difference between the HMO reimbursed amount and the actual charges that might accrue.

The programmable hearing aid that "Barney" selects to fit the patient's reduced hearing exceeds the agreed-on limit for a single hearing aid by nearly $400. What are "Barney's" options? Here are some:

A. Honor the contract and lose money.
B. Renegotiate the contract in light of new technology.
C. Leave the choice to the patient after explaining the problem.
D. Ask for an exception to the contract.
E. Dispense the hearing aid that the HMO will pay for, not the programmable one, and tell the patient why.
F. Refer the patient to another audiologist for the aid and share in the profit.

---

[2] "Ginger" is. Material for the Yellow Pages was sent in months before it appeared. She had no right to list her *anticipated* qualifications. So is the supervisor for not signing the CFY form.

    G. Ask the patient to donate the difference to the hospital's "needy sick fund."

    H. Run up more service charges to cover the uncovered cost of the hearing aid.

Some of the choices are clearly unethical. If "Barney" is reported to an ethics committee for following one of the alleged unethical choices, diversity would not be an acceptable explanation. If there is diversity in "Barney's" practice, it is self-inflicted. No special exceptions to the code can be imposed in this instance. Other choices presented are obviously ethical, but clearly not good business. That, of course, is the ethics dilemma that arises between business choices and the principles of practicing as a member of a profession.

There is yet another concern raised by the current practice of some health care providers. This is the question, for example, of whether an HMO is responsible for causing practitioners to violate ethics codes by negotiating services contracts that limit the care a professional can provide. Answers to that question may not help "Barney" at this stage, but the quandary is worthy of consideration by those who negotiate professional service agreements. Probably "Barney's" best option is to ask for an exception (D) and also try to renegotiate the contract (B).

Case 4: The 8-Karat Golden Rule

Let's assume two weeks have passed since Case 4, and another HMO hearing aid candidate comes to "Barney" for service. No programmable hearing aids are considered for the client because no settlement has been reached in the first "Barney Smith" matter, although this patient is as good a candidate for a programmable device as was the first patient. This time "Barney" recommends and sells another type of instrument.

The next day the patient calls and says, "I met a guy at a party last night who has one of those programmable hearing aids. How come that wasn't tried on me?" "Barney" tells him the truth, and he claims "Barney" is unethical and reports him to the association's ethics committee. Is Barney unethical? What might the ethics committee do?

The problem is not simple because of the terms of the contract that the audiologist negotiated. It is a mixed situation for that reason and because the audiologist, perhaps, provided less than quality service. If the contract is being renegotiated there is the chance that an ethics committee will await the outcome before rendering a decision. The fact remains, nonetheless, that the audiologist did provide a lesser service to the second patient and this may be a minimally sanctionable conduct.

There is also the chance that the committee will cite the audiologist for not referring the patient for something that he could not provide, as required by the code. The welfare of the patient has not been held paramount. The committee could also correspond with the HMO indicating the ethics concern, thus supporting the need for a contract amendment. A letter of this nature would not, however, relieve the audiologist from possible citation.

REGISTERING A COMPLAINT

The best way to file a complaint of ethical impropriety against a member of a professional association is most often by letter. This is the case with the American Academy of Audiology, as an example (AAA, 1991). The letter should state the alleged impropriety clearly, with as much factual information included as possible. It is not necessary to cite the section of the code violated. The ethics committee will eventually determine that. The letter must be signed, but initially is held as a confidential document by the committee. The committee classifies the letter writer as the "claimant." The individual reported is referred to as the "respondent." It is perfectly acceptable for more than one person to sign a letter of complaint.

On receipt of the complaint the committee should acknowledge receipt to the claimant and make an initial determination of whether the reported action is a probable ethics matter that falls within their jurisdiction. The committee in some associations requests that the claimant agree to be made known to the respondent, although this is not always a necessary requirement of ethics committees. The dogma that the accused has the right to know an accuser is precedent. ASHA and AAA do make such a request, however.

Once the committee determines that an alleged incident is actionable and in their jurisdiction, the respondent is notified of the allegation received by the committee. The accuser is **not** made known to the respondent at this time. The respondent is asked to provide a detailed explanation of the incident reported—that is, to defend the alleged impropriety. An ethics committee may at the same time correspond with others involved in the reported incident in an effort to obtain as much factual information as possible to judge the allegation.

THE INITIAL DETERMINATION

Following receipt of all the information pertaining to the case the committee discusses the issues as a group. A determination of guilt or

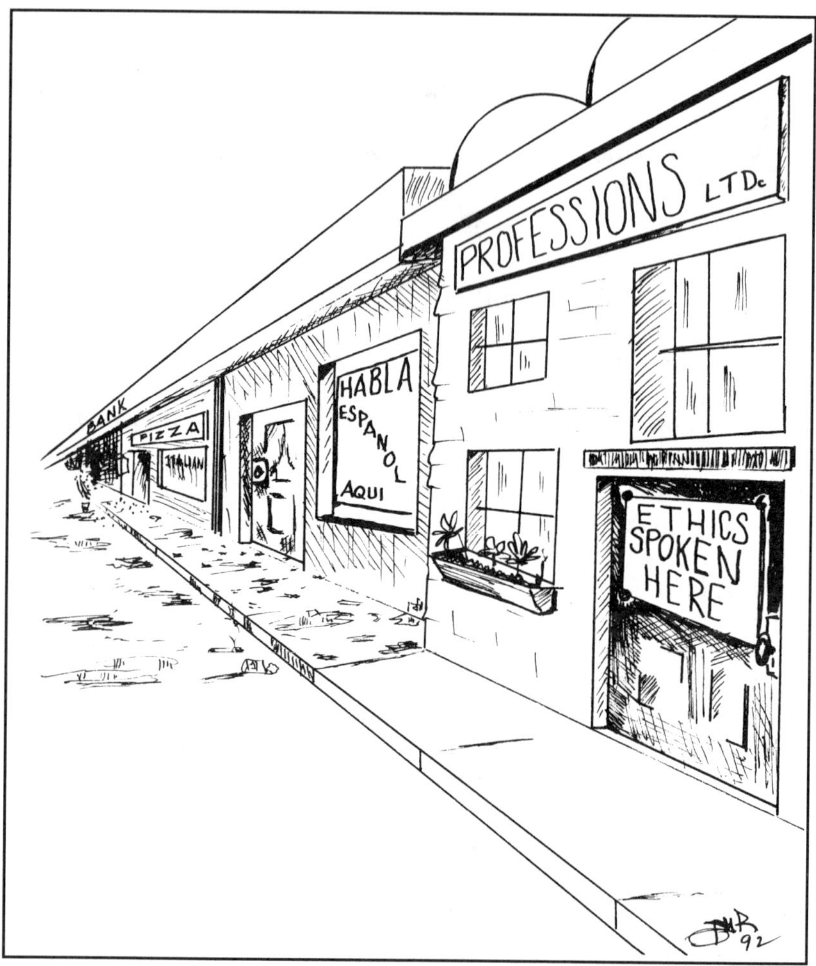

innocence is reached and a sanction assigned. The respondent is noti-fied of the finding. In ASHA this finding is called "the initial determi-nation" (ASHA, 1991). It allows the respondent to seek what ASHA's ethics board refers to as "a further consideration hearing."

The Further Consideration Hearing

Essentially the further consideration hearing adds an informal step to "due process" by providing an opportunity for the respondent to clarify misunderstandings, misinterpretations, or make a plea for a lesser sanction.

ASHA's ethics board allows this further consideration hearing to be conducted in person, or by telephone, with or without legal representation present. Following the further consideration hearing, the committee either reaffirms the initial determination, or makes an appropriate adjustment in the finding, based on the further consideration hearing.

The offering of a further consideration hearing certainly goes beyond what is usually required of an ethics committee and offers the respondent an added opportunity to obtain release from a finding of an ethics infraction. The step precedes the right of formal appeal, which the respondent also has. Formal appeal is also part of due process, but it is only acceptable as an option if the respondent can show a factual error in the procedure of the ethics committee, or in the degree of sanction in relation to the ethics violation. Formal appeals cannot be filed merely because the respondent does not agree with the committee's determination. Respondents rarely agree with the finding of an ethics committee, unless, of course, they are exonerated. Formal appeals are heard before a different body than the ethics committee. In ASHA this is the Council on Professional Ethics (COPE). The finding of COPE is final.

The disadvantage of a further consideration hearing is that it lengthens the time a case is in process—sometimes substantially. When an alleged violation clearly impacts the quality of service provided by the respondent an ethics committee has the right to require the respondent to "cease and desist" from the alleged unethical conduct until a committee determination is reached. Obviously this can have a negative effect on a respondent's practice, and the effect can be made worse by the length of time required for a further consideration hearing.

The AAA does not provide for a further consideration hearing, but the association does allow an appeal of ethics committee findings. The appeal must be based on procedural errors or excessive sanctions not suited to the infraction. Appeals are heard by the Executive Committee of the Academy and their determination is final.

In all matters related to ethics committee case deliberations, confidentiality is of the utmost importance during processing. Claimants and respondents have a right to privacy and that right is respected by ethics committees. That is not to imply that ethics committees do not share information with other committees of other associations. Sometimes they do. When they do, however, confidentiality is maintained between and among the committees.

Obviously the business of an ethics committee and those deciding appeals is a serious undertaking. The groups hold in their hands the welfare of professional practitioners as well as the public image of the association they represent. Ethics committees keep the welfare of claimants and respondents paramount, but there is also the obligation to perform the duties of the committee to the best of their ability.

It is fairly clear (*Shulman v. The Washington Hospital Center*, 1963; *Withrow v. Larkin*, 1975) that due process is not violated when the same ethics body functions in both investigative and decision-making roles. In *Withrow v. Larkin*, however, the Supreme court did warn that although the mere exposure to evidence is not sufficient in itself to impugn the fairness of board members, nevertheless, "we should be alert to the possibilities of bias that may lurk in the way particular procedures actually work in practice."

Matters of professional ethics may indeed require a change driven by moral, economic, and humanistic issues. But that change may actually tighten rather than relax principles. Similarly, matters of jurisdiction, diversity, and the rules by which professions provide their service will continue to be deliberated by those entrusted with the formulation, interpretation, and monitoring of ethics codes for some time to come. Those issues, too, may come to rest in tougher standards and a longer reach. Whatever the future holds concerning jurisdiction and diversity, at least for now it appears best to play by the rules that are in now existence.

5

Beware the Bearer of Gifts

Progress, far from consisting in change, depends on retentiveness.
Those who cannot remember the past are condemned to fulfill it.
(Santayana)

Marketing strategies as practiced by commercial enterprises are well thought out plans designed to profit a particular business. The techniques are varied and function in a kaleidoscope of ways on the consumer. In general, marketing is a business ethics means of attracting customers, but sometimes the methods used give rise to the concern of professional organizations.

Marketing techniques as practiced by large commercial industries are far too expensive for smaller businesses to undertake. Many small industries, as a matter of fact, believe the large conglomerates take unfair marketing advantage of the small companies. Marketing is unfamiliar territory to professions, although some professions today tend to place more emphasis on the techniques and skills of marketing a private practice than ever before. The influences that marketing has, both good and less than good, on the professions is an important issue to the ethics of a profession.

EFFECTS OF MARKETING ON THE PROFESSIONS

Because marketing expenses increase the cost of goods to users, the U.S. government examines the marketing practices of large companies from which goods or services are purchased. For example, as reported in the *Washington Post* (November, 1990) the use of gifts and other marketing strategies by some pharmaceutical manufacturing companies was under heavy criticism in 1990 by the Senate Labor and Human Resources Committee headed by Senator Edward Kennedy. The government's interest obviously stemmed from the high cost of medicines in Medicare—a cost continuing to escalate. The Senate Committee was asking hard questions about relationships between commercial makers and movers of prescriptive medicines and the physicians prescribing them. And the Legislature was doing it publicly.

A disabling tactic was mounted by the American Medical Association in December of 1990, however, in an attempt to divert apparent negative publicity according to a story in the *Washington Post* (Weiss,1990). At that time the AMA's House of Delegates adopted, without dissent, a set of ethical guidelines proposed by its Council on Ethical and Judicial Affairs (American Medical Association, 1991). Among other prohibitions, the AMA guidelines now judge unethical the acceptance of subsidized vacations, outright cash gifts, or cash to pay for travel expenses to conferences/seminars, CEU-touted events, and lavish meals and entertainment from pharmaceutical companies.

These and other marketing practices have been liberally applied over the years to influence physicians' drug-prescribing decisions. Adoption of the guidelines now incorporated into the AMA's Code of Ethics for the Medical Profession follows one year of deliberations. The guidelines became effective January 1, 1991.

The 100-plus member Pharmaceutical Manufacturers Association (PMA) adopted the same guidelines two days after the AMA acceptance.

True, many gifts given to physicians by companies in the pharmaceutical and medical device and equipment industries serve an important and socially beneficial function. Companies have, for example, long provided funds for educational seminars and conferences. However, there has been growing concern about certain gifts from industry to physicians. Some gifts that reflect the customary practices of certain industries may not be consistent with the principles of medical ethics, and to avoid the acceptance of inappropriate gifts, physicians are now required to comply with the following guidelines to their Code of Ethics:

> <> Any gifts accepted by physicians individually should primarily entail a benefit to patients and should not be of substantial value. Accordingly, textbooks, modest meals, and other gifts are appropriate if they serve a genuine educational function. Cash payments should not be accepted.

<> Individual gifts of minimal value are permissible as long as the gifts are related to the physician's work (e.g., pens, notepads).

<> Subsidies to underwrite the costs of continuing medical education conferences or professional meetings can contribute to the improvement of patient care and are therefore permissible. Since the giving of a subsidy directly to a physician by a company's sales representative may create a relationship that could influence the use of the company's products, any subsidy should be accepted by the conference's sponsor who, in turn, can use the money to reduce the conference's registration fee. Payments to defray the costs of a conference should not be accepted directly from the company by physicians who are attending the conference.

<> Subsidies should not be accepted directly or indirectly to pay for the cost of travel, lodging or other personal expenses of physicians in attendance, nor should subsidies be accepted to compensate for physicians' time. Subsidies for hospitality should not be accepted outside of modest meals or social events that are held as part of a conference or meeting. It is permissible for faculty at conferences or meetings to accept honoraria and to accept reimbursement for reasonable travel, lodging and meal expenses. It is also appropriate for consultants who provide genuine services to receive reasonable compensation and reimbursement for travel, lodging and meal expense. Token consulting and advisory arrangements can not be used to justify the compensation of physicians for their time or their travel, lodging, and other out-of-pocket expenses.

<> Scholarship or other special funds to permit medical students, residents, and fellows to attend carefully selected educational conferences may be permissible as long as the selection of students, residents, or fellows who will receive the funds is made by the academic or training institution.

<> No gifts should be accepted if there are strings attached. For example, physicians should not accept gifts if they are given in relation to the physician's prescribing practices. In addition, when companies underwrite medical conferences or lectures other than their own, responsibility for and control over the selection and content, faculty, educational methods, and materials should belong to the organizers of the conferences or lectures.

Adoption of these guidelines preceded by one week a two-day session of hearings conducted by Kennedy and the Labor and Human Resources Committee. During testimony by physicians and former pharmaceutical company executives, extravagant marketing practices were revealed, including:

1. Sending physicians and their spouses on all-expense paid trips to Acapulco, Palm Springs, Monte Carlo for "educa-

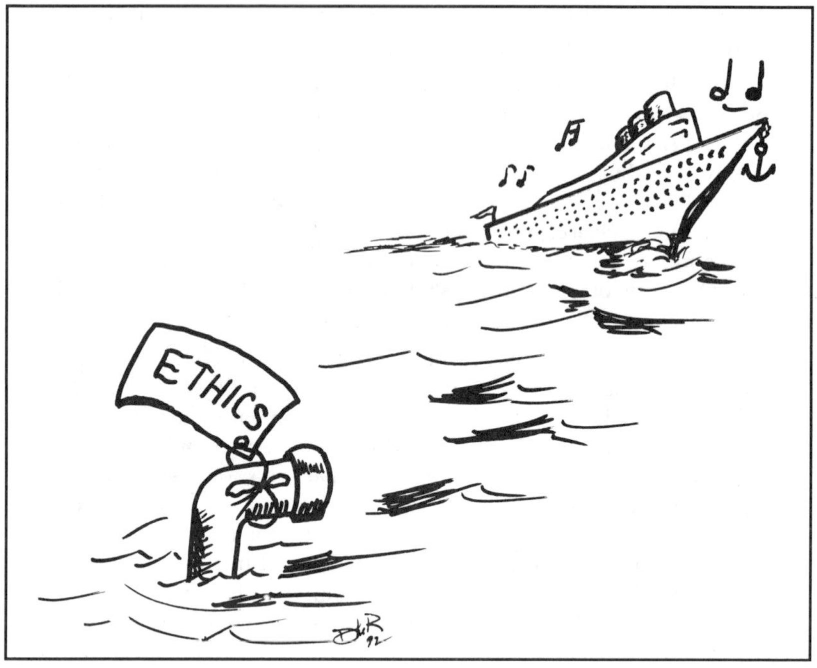

tional" symposia—events that cost the company (and ultimately the consumer) more than half a million dollars each...

2. Offering physicians $1,200 to prescribe an expensive antibiotic to 20 patients in a "clinical study." The study was funded by the marketing division of the pharmaceutical company and involved physicians providing data that were essentially demographic in nature. The cost of therapy purchased by 20 patients for the common course of the medication would bring the company sales of $11,400...

3. Awarding airline frequent flyer miles for prescriptions written...

4. Offering a physician $100 for simply reading a company's literature that encouraged prescribing a highly toxic drug for a use that was not approved by the Food and Drug Administration...

Of particular interest is that the same companies bestowing gifts on physicians restrict their own employees from accepting any type of gratuity having a value greater than $5. Their reasoning is sound: The risk of influence is greater than any benefit to the company.

Although United States Senator Ted Kennedy has acknowledged in television interviews that physicians who accept lavish gifts are jeopardizing their objectivity and compromising the trust of their patients, his deepest concern is that the consumer finances these marketing practices, which deliver no health benefit, through higher drug prices. Drug prices, for example, escalated 88% from 1981 to 1988. General price inflation during the same period was 28%, according to Kennedy in the *Washington Post* (November, 1990) citing statistics appearing in an unspecified *Fortune* magazine survey.

It is surprising to the average citizen, and apparent bad business practice to some corporate thinkers, that the pharmaceutical industry would voluntarily give up marketing practices that bolster their profits. These successful practices have been in place for decades. The highly competitive industry is also among the most profitable in the United States, with a 13% return on sales in 1989. At least $5 billion of their total $32.4 billion sales was spent on marketing—more than $8,000 per physician in the United States in 1989.

The lingering concern, of course, is for the long-long-term effect on consumer (and therefore government) costs for medication. Additionally, the AMA may be wondering about sustained affect publicity surrounding the Senate hearings may have on the traditional public trust in a physician's objectivity. Other professions are watching carefully for a potential spillover that could eventually jeopardize health care reimbursement dollars from fiscal intermediaries.

Although Medicare provides no reimbursement to audiologists for hearing aids or related services, for example, there still may be reason for audiologists to be concerned. An important question involves the parallels, if any, to be found with present-day relationships between hearing aid/equipment manufacturers and audiologists and the PMA-physician relationship scrutinized by the government. Conceivably the time has come for all professional associations to be at least wary of those who bear gifts. The potential for conflict of interest is high.

CONFLICTS OF INTEREST

Distinguishing among sources of conflicts of interest is not easy. Professional practitioners tend to overlook conflicts, or gloss through them with an attitude of, "I would never do a thing like that. I care too much for those I serve." But that attitude is simply not enough. If it were, there would be no need for a code of conduct in any profession and Hippocrates and all those following have deliberated in vain.

Commercial relationships between practitioners and product providers seems to be the greatest single source of potential conflict of interest arrangements. There are others, however, such as practitioner ownership in a commercial venture with the potential for abuse; compensation systems based on quotas; selling the product prescribed; fee splitting; contractual group practice arrangements, and so on. Nearly all have something to do with the economics of a professional practice. Nearly all, at least on the surface, oppose the intent of a code of ethics of a profession. That is not to say, however, that many apparent conflicts cannot be managed in a way that is satisfactory to professional conduct.

The underlying principle is that practitioners must take clear and definite steps to prevent conflicts of interest and to avoid the appearance of conflicts of interest. This position is derived from the tradition that a professional's duty is to act primarily for another's benefit in matters pertaining to the professional's area of expertise. Further, the ethical issue for the practitioner should always be to assure, insofar as possible, that when the inevitable conflicts do occur they should be resolved at minimum not only to comply with the law and public policy, but more often than not conflicts should also be settled in favor of the consumer of professional service.

Individual health field practitioners may choose the strictest personal moral code, of course, such as totally avoiding financial interests in facilities, products, devices, and so forth that may be used in the provision of health care services. In many professions that is not a viable option. Nevertheless, a middle ground should be permissible as long as priority is placed on the welfare of the receiver of services. That's the keystone of professional ethics in relateship to conflicts of interest.

In medicine, the belief that financial interest should not interfere with the physician's medical judgments on behalf of the patient is ancient. It is best exemplified in Maimonides' prayer (Etziony, 1973):

> Do not allow thirst for profit, ambition for renown and admiration, to interfere with my profession for these are the enemies of truth and can lead me astray in the great task of attending to the welfare of Your creatures. (p. 262)

In 1986, B. H. Gray, in a book entitled *For Profit Enterprise in Health Care* indicated that all compensations in the professions, from fee-for-service to capitation or salary present some undesirable incentives for providing too many services or too few. But no system will work without some degree of integrity, decency, and ethical commitment on the part of professionals. Inevitably, some underlying professionalism must be presumed that will constrain unadulterated self-interest.

The solution is not to find a set of incentives that is beyond criticism, but to seek arrangements that encourage professional functioning in the highest sense of that term. As previously discussed, certain changes that are occurring in an increasingly entrepreneurial health care system can quickly undermine patients' trust in, for example, their physician and society's trust in the professions. For those who believe professionalism is an essential element in ensuring, wherever possible, the quality of health care, this becomes an important concern.

An interesting opinion was published by the AMA Council on Ethical and Judicial Affairs (1986) on physician dispensing of drugs or devices to patients for profit. Deliberation of the situation revolved around (A) public policy, which in several states prohibits physicians from dispensing if there is exploitation of the patient, but permits it if there is disclosure and patient choice, and (B) prescription of a drug or use of a device produced by a company in which the practitioner holds publicly traded stock, the profits and losses of which are determined by total market forces, compared to the situation whereby the practitioner's dispensing creates a conflict of interest if the prescribed items are available through normal channels. In other words, the matter of personal gain is less important when the value of that gain (loss) results from public interest in the stock of the company.

The recommendations from the council suggest that, although there are circumstances in which physicians may ethically engage in the dispensing of drugs, devices, or other products, physicians are urged to avoid regular dispensing of products when the needs of the patient can be met by local pharmacies or suppliers.

Another source of possible conflict of interest involves the situation where the professional refers a patient to a facility or service owned in whole or in part by the professional. It is acceptable that, for example, a physician may own or operate a pharmacy if there is no resulting exploitation of patients. The practitioner (in the case of the pharmacy) is required to (American Medical Association, 1981) :

1. Disclose personal ownership interest in the pharmacy;
2. Prescribe only that quantity of drug reasonably required for the patient's condition;
3. Comply with all applicable laws, including those that restrict referral to one's own facility;
4. Provide a written prescription to allow the patient a choice of having it filled elsewhere; and
5. Make alternative arrangements for the care of the patient if the physician's commercial interest conflicts so greatly with the best interest of the patient as to be incompatible.

Public policy, as reflected in various statutes, ranges from total prohibition of referral to the practitioner's business interest, through the middle ground of requiring disclosure as described immediately above to no restrictions of any kind. One might wonder if there is a lesson to be learned here for otolaryngology practices that hold a separate corporation or business dedicated to audiology, vestibular, electrophysiologic measurements, or the sale of hearing aids.

The ethical dilemma requires determination of what degree of financial interest creates a possible conflict of interest with the patient's best interests. If the practitioner is the sole owner of the entity to which patients are referred and if the practitioner's income is dependent on the level or degree of ownership, there is conflict of interest. Failure to disclose would be deceitful.

Interesting at this point for the ethics in the fields of speech-language pathology and audiology is the relationship that some otolaryngologists have with speech and hearing persons who either:

A. Work as an employee in the office;

B. Work as a partner in the office;

C. Manage a hearing/speech/balance center owned by the physician; or

D. Provide hearing aid dispensing services as an outside contractor, but in the physician's office.

It appears that the constraints previously mentioned are placed on the ethics of the physician only. Neither the ASHA nor the AAA directly address issues of this nature in their codes of ethics. There has been no need for it in the past. However, business opportunities are presented to professional practices today with increasing frequency, and to some practitioners the chance is too good to ignore. Perhaps, if financially cooperative work settings for audiologists and speech-language pathologists continue to increase, the ethics codes of their professional associations will need to reflect sensitivity to the need for a specific guideline in the area of business ownership and so forth.

Fee splitting is yet another area for consideration and a particularly difficult one because of the increase in newly devised business arrangements. Again, according to the ethics of the American College of Physicians (1984) and the AMA (1991) a physician may not accept payment of any kind, in any form, from any source, such as pharmaceutical companies, pharmacists, optical companies, or the manufacturers of medical appliances or devices, for prescribing or referring a patient for the purchase of medicines, glasses, or appliances. In each case the payment would violate the requirement that the practitioner has to deal honestly with the patient and with colleagues. The patient relies on the advice of the professional, and the restrictions placed on medical practitioners should serve as a strong guidepost for other professional health care workers.

This type of restriction on physicians comes close to a situation that most audiologists in private practice fear. That is, what are the ethical risks taken when audiologists are involved in the various discount purchase schemes or purchase incentive programs hosted by manufacturers of products used by audiologists in a practice. There is no doubt that risks are taken; there is, at the very least, the *appearance* of a conflict of interest. Whether an actual violation of the code for audiologists/speech-language pathologists actually occurs depends, obviously, on specific circumstances of a given incident.

Optometrists, to whom audiologists are most often likened, are denied by Section III C of the Code of Ethics and Standards of Conduct of the American Optometric Association (1976) from accepting rebates on prescriptions, lenses, or optical appliances used in the practice of optometry. No such specifically worded restriction is placed on audiologists in the ASHA or AAA Codes, although cautions on apparent conflicts of interest seek to control the lure of the strong marketing tactics of big business.

Financial rewards to professionals for the referral of patients or for *not* referring patients, instances of fee-splitting, proprietary ownership, and the like can all have, at least, the appearance of impropriety and can undermine the public's confidence in the profession. Professional decisions must be based in the best interests of the person served, and not in the self-interest of the provider.

SOME STATE STATUTES

The following references to selected state statutes and opinions of state attorneys general are included as illustrations of various public policy approaches to potential conflict of interest situations. This is not intended as a comprehensive review of the law on the subject, but rather as an example of the diversity existing at the state level. The practice of audiology/speech-language pathology, although not mentioned specifically in any of the statutes, could easily be addressed in most of them.

A Florida statute (1981) provides that the following are grounds for disciplinary action against professional practitioners:

> Exercising influence on the patient or client in such a manner as to exploit the patient or client for financial gain of the [professional] ... which shall include but not be limited to the promoting or selling of services or goods, appliances, or drugs and the promoting

or advertising on any prescription form of a community pharmacy unless the form shall also state "this prescription may be filled at any pharmacy of your choice."

An Illinois statute (1986) provides that the promotion or sale of drugs, devices, appliance, or goods "provided for a patient in such a manner as to exploit the patient" ... [provides] "the basis for disciplinary action."

An opinion of the Missouri attorney general (1982) indicates that, "a physician who requires that a patient accept drugs dispensed by the physician and refuses to provide the patient ... [free choice] ... may be in violation of the Missouri Antitrust Law."

Rhode Island (1985) defines punishable unprofessional conduct to include "any promotion by a physician ... of the sale of" [product] "in a manner to exploit the patient for the financial gain of the" [practitioner].

A Texas statute (Roeder & Shimberg, 1986) allows a licensed physician to supply the needs of patients with anything necessary, but a physician is "not permitted to operate a retail pharmacy store without first complying with the Texas Pharmacy Act."

A Virginia statute (Corbett v. D'Allesandro 1985) provides that the following constitutes unprofessional conduct:

> Being a practitioner in the healing arts who may lawfully dispense, administer, or prescribe medicines, or drugs, and not being the holder of a certificate of registration to practice pharmacy, engages in selling medicine, drugs, eyeglasses, or medical appliances or devices to his [sic] own patients either for his [sic] own convenience, or for the purpose of supplementing his [sic] income, provided, however, that the dispensing of contact lenses by a practitioner to [his] own patients shall not be deemed to be for the practitioner's own convenience or for the purpose of supplementing his [sic] income.

A Michigan attorney general's opinion (*Natanson v. Kline*, 1979) provides that "violation of the prohibition against a licensed health professional having a financial interest in a clinical laboratory is not avoided by disclosure to the individual being directed or required to obtain a service, drug, device, treatment, or procedure."

Although the many state statutes are directed specifically at the licensed medical practitioner, the laws offer a model against which the professional practices of everyone providing health care services can be measured.

CONFLICTS OF INTEREST IN RESEARCH

The avoidance of real or perceived conflict of interest in clinical research is yet another ethics dilemma. Ethics control in research is imperative if the research community is to protect objectivity, maintain individual and institutional integrity, and present an image of these qualities to the outside world. The task is difficult in part because of the paucity of objective information about what constitutes ethical behavior in the research setting. Surely one of the key areas at risk is the economic conflicts of interest in research center–industry research collaboration situations.

Unfortunately, conflict of interest in clinical research defies simple definition: one researcher's conflict of interest may be another's mutually beneficial working relationship, indicates Palca (1989). Institutional Review Boards (IRBs) monitor the conduct of researchers as one of their responsibilities. Conflict of interest must be clearly distinguished from scientific misconduct. The generally accepted patterns that constitute misconduct in science include plagiarism, deception, and falsification and/or fabrication of data. Scientific misconduct compromises the integrity of the scientific process. Conflict of interest presents a distinct subset of issues.

The most suitable working definition is that a conflict of interest is a dynamic tension between the private interests and the official responsibilities of a person in a position of trust.

Although conflicts of interest are inherent in any research relationship, perhaps the most important area in which conflict may arise is when a researcher enters into a financial arrangement with a profit-making corporation. However, the general norms of scientific behavior, including intellectual honesty and objectivity, reasonable doubt, etc., are not necessarily compromised when a conflict of interest does arise.

Clinical trials involving a specific product are typically funded by industry, with researchers pursuing questions of basic biologic processes traditionally not finding much research support except from the federal government. Although industry support for research has risen sharply in recent years according to Hoppin (1987), it still represents only about 5% of the total external funding received by research universities. University-based research in biotechnology, however, receives from 16% to 24% of its support from industry (Blumenthal, 1986).

Estimates indicate that nearly half of all biotechnology firms support research in universities (AMA White Paper, 1988), and that 90 of the top 100 universities conducting biotech research receive financial support from industrial sources. Moreover, university faculty are employed as consultants by 90% of the biotech companies, and nearly 50% of faculty researchers in biotechnology serve as consultants to industry. These types of arrangements are important to the survival of both industry and academia, as the research environment, like the clinical environment, becomes increasingly competitive.

The risks for possible conflict of interest for the investigator include:

- Restrictions imposed by the sponsor on publication or use of research findings;
- Pressures to emphasize commercial ventures at the expense of patient care;
- Reductions in the amount of time available for clinical duties;
- Increased pressures to disseminate only those results that are of benefit to the corporation; and
- Potential cost-shifting to patients.

Problems may arise when the researcher has a direct financial interest in the research program or in the outcome of a project. In perhaps the most prominent case, an ophthalmologist studied an experimental eye ointment while owning in excess of 50,000 shares of stock in the company that was formed to market the product (Culliton, 1988). Investigations revealed that the ophthalmologist made unauthorized modification to a study and minimized negative findings before selling his stock at a profit (Leary, 1989).

As with other possible violations of a professional code of ethics, it is extremely important in the research milieu that a separation be made between real problems and the *perception* of a conflict of interest. Ethics guidelines for clinical researchers facing economic conflicts of interest ultimately turn on two principles:

- First, researchers may ethically share in the economic rewards of their efforts.
- Second, there must be clear evidence that potential sources of bias in research have been eliminated to the extent possible.

CONFLICTS OF INTEREST AMONG LAY WORKERS

Workers other than the pure professionals are obviously more vulnerable to conflicts of interest. Most would like to change that level of susceptibility, either for themselves or the fields they represent. Most are not willing to divest themselves of those aspects of their work effort that result in conflicts of interest.

Consider the current situation with financial planners—that group of salespeople who are skilled at rendering advice concerning what to do with *your* money. They want respect, and they figure the best way to get it is to have some uniform standards of conduct as, they say, do doctors and lawyers.

The financial planners are having a tough time, though, deciding how rigid those standards should be. This is especially true when it comes to the sensitive subject of whether to disclose the big commissions many planners earn when they sell investment products. The whole issue of trying to develop a code of conduct shatters when self-interest is at the root.

The topic of commissions highlights the fundamental conflict of interest facing the financial planning industry: While all planners typically charge a fee to evaluate a person's finances and make recommendations, many get the bulk of their income from product commissions. The hard questions that need answers before financial planners can come to grips with standards of conduct equal to those of professional associations are: Should planners be required to place clients' interests ahead of their own? Should planners be required to solve clients' problems through financial recommendations that might not generate high commissions? Should planners be required to disclose the amount of commission on each item recommended?

Among organizations interested in making financial planners more respectable in the eyes of the public there is even a suggestion to use the word "fiduciary," a legal term that denotes obligation, as in "the financial planner has a fiduciary responsibility to put the interests of the client first and foremost." Some call this intent a legal nightmare that will induce every disgruntled client to sue. Perhaps so, but that may be the cost of acquiring or improving public trust, and the question merely becomes one of how much a business is willing to pay to have a code of ethics and put self-interest in second place.

Federal, state, and local governments are also looking at the ethics of how they do what they do, particularly regarding areas of potential conflict of interest. Although not professionals in the traditional definition of the word, politicians feel uncomfortable with situations where ethics officers monitor the ethics of the same people who appoint them.

To lessen potential for conflicts of interest among state employees, most state ethics laws follow a general trend of prohibiting staff employees and officials from:

1. Participating in an official capacity in activities where they, or relatives, have an interest;
2. Serving in any employment relationship that would impair impartiality or independence of judgment;
3. Soliciting or accepting gifts from anyone who ever engaged in an activity regulated by the state.

Some states also have an ethics law requiring employees to complete a form every year listing gifts received in excess of $50.

Conflicts of interest appear in an apparent high percentage of personal income producing endeavors. Surprising, though, is that in those fields where self-interest has always been obvious, there is increasing enthusiasm for controlling sources of possible conflict of interest. Not surprising is the loss of that enthusiasm when the business/trade organizations become aware of the price to be paid to gain the public trust. The professions, at least for now, are still willing to invest in whatever it takes to keep the welfare of the consumer of professional services uppermost.

MITIGATING CONFLICTS

If professions are to continue to deserve the public trust, the matter of apparent conflicts of interest must be dealt with not only in the interests of the consumer, but to the satisfaction of the professional association facing the dilemma. The AMA has apparently met the challenge head-on, albeit that it took a Senate investigating committee to prod them into making an overt adjustment in their practices and their relationships with pharmaceutical manufacturers. The commercial relationship between manufacturers and practitioners in speech-language pathology may not be as important to the federal government as the relationship between the medical profession and the commercial providers of goods required for the practice of medicine, but it, at least, requires self-awareness that practitioners may be subject to criticism.

There is no ethics argument with the fact that professions must have the goods provided by commercial entities, and that a solid relationship must exist between the parties in order to obtain the best service for the consumer. Moreover, no ethics committee can dispute, and no practitioner should doubt, that the control of any relationship between commercial organizations and professionals rests squarely with the professional.

When that control slips out of the hands of the practitioner, when the balance shifts, or *appears* to shift, to lay rather than professional control then ethics monitors raise their antennae. The situation poses a great risk that the practitioner's self-interest will replace the profession's interest in the welfare of the consumer. The risk to the profession should always be assumed greater than the promised benefit.

It is far better for professional associations to recognize the potential conflicts of interest posed by commercial relationships and to adjust their practices before official inquiries are mounted into the practices of the association. Such matters are always settled more agreeably away from the heat of battle, rather than at the time of inquiry. Every professional has an obligation to attend to those behaviors that have the appearance of a conflict of interest. It is the ethical thing to do.

6

Balancing the Ethics of a Profession and a Business

Nobody ever did anything foolish except from strong principle.
(Lord David Cecil)

One of the difficult tasks associated with being a professional in today's venue is to remain sensitive to the features that distinguish a profession from a business or a trade. Once distinguished, those distinctive attributes must be protected if professions are to survive as professions and not simply as work settings engaged in the sale of health care and a variety of health care products.

It is unfortunate, but true that the matter of ethics is usually raised *after* a particular infraction has occurred rather than having been considered before a specific conduct is undertaken. In similar fashion, concern for professional ethics is seldom raised by commercial enterprises in their relations with the professions. Recall the swiftness of the Pharmaceutical Manufacturers' Association to agree and comply with the guidelines supported by the AMA *after* the Senate hearings exposed questionable marketing habits. If ethics concerns aren't dealt with by the professional participators, they are probably not brought out at all, and conduct continues unchallenged for so long that it is falsely assumed to be acceptable behavior. It is the responsibility of the professional to guide the behavior between the profession and industry.

But what about circumstances where the professional and the entrepreneur is the same person who must manage a professional practice as a business, or a business in the model of a professional practice? Even though the two endeavors seem mutually exclusive, there must be room for coexistence—a balance of sorts. Medicine does it. Dentistry does it. Psychology does it, as do all other professions.

The way to success, the balance of sorts, must allow the coexistence to be dominated by professionalism not entrepreneurship. Professionals must be aware of the variety of issues that have an impact on a profession as well as a business, and must maintain an ethics attitude and practice to assure that professions preserve the trust afforded them by the consuming public. Not to do so emphatically is to dilute the professionalism the public expects.

THE ISSUES

With continued growth in the number of private practicing audiologists and speech-language pathologists the maintenance of a conscious distinction between the values held by professionals and the motives embraced by business persons becomes crucial to their fields' preservation as professions. The primary reason for this is, in the case of audiology, that the practice depends heavily on the sale of hearing aids to be financially successful. The prescription of product, and the sale of the same product by the one who prescribes it leaves a thin veil between the pathways of a business and a profession.

Many times the public is unable to discern the veil and instead believes the vendor of product and the professional health care service provider are the same person. At times they are. But the public must be able to see the difference between the caregiver who is motivated by self-interest and the professional who keeps the welfare of the person served paramount.

Although a clear demarcation between professions and businesses is preferable, there is also an obvious connection between the two that cannot be ignored, and that becomes most apparent in the maintenance of nearly all private professional practices engaging in product sales—audiology, optometry, ophthalmology, otolaryngology, dentistry, and the like. The ingredient important for the perpetuation of both the business and professional aspects of practice is *need*. Professional practices need commercial industry for the supply of quality goods used in the management of persons treated by the professions. Commercial industries need the professional practitioner to sell the manufactured goods in large amount. Reliance of one entity on the other is a reality.

The ethics of professions indicates that the welfare of the person served is of primary concern; and state further not to overtreat, not to undertreat, to refer if you cannot treat, and so on—self-interest is *not* the motivating force. The ethics of businesses indicate basically that one should do unto others; they imply, for example, not to overcharge, not to undercharge, not to lie about the product, and so on—self-interest *is* the motivating force.

When the practice of professionals involves the sale of a product the practice becomes a business. At least for that time, the professional serves two masters—the welfare of the patient and the success of the business. It is said that no one can serve two masters, for soon one master is loved and the other is hated. The paradox created by the reliance of professions on industry and vice versa, is difficult to resolve because many practitioners vacillate between wanting the respectability of a professional and the flexibility of an entrepreneur.

Audiologists, for example, are quick to point out that as professionals they would only do what is best for the welfare of those entrusted to their care. As professionals they wouldn't undertake a treatment, or sell a product for any reason other than the patient's good, and they don't need an ethics statement to govern that behavior. That's what they say. Why should it be doubted?

Industry people are equally quick to indicate that they are always trying to provide the best commodity through the practitioner for the consumer's welfare. As product representatives they wouldn't convince anyone to purchase a product that wasn't the best. That would not be good business and it would not perpetuate a steady stream of customers. That's what they say. Why should it be doubted? Individuals who may be both audiologist and entrepreneur find themselves in a difficult position. One requiring a choice.

These altruistic convictions may all be true. What is also true, however, is that, for some reason, neither the professionals nor the industry workers want to see published standards in the form of a code of ethics publicizing those convictions to the consumer—thereby preserving one of the distinguishing ethical characteristics of a profession.

The reasons for their objections are not clear. Logically it would seem that if each is already holding the welfare of their patients and customers paramount, that is, everyone is functioning in compliance with a professional code of ethics, then stating the standards should have no effect on their practice. Conversely, if they are marching to the drumbeat of self-interest, it is likely that some practice procedures would violate the ethics of the profession.

Some audiologists seem to view restrictive statements such as professional ethics codes as paternalistic, a demonstration that their professional association has no trust in their judgment. Ethics, they seem to feel, is something that *is*, not something that has to be specified. They say they know right from wrong. But we all do, most of the time. At least most people don't have much trouble in separating what's *absolutely* right from what is absolutely wrong.

Generally, nobody wants to get into a lengthy discussion about what is honest or fair, what is ethical and what is unethical.

Nobody Is Perfect

Pobody's nerfect, and most people feel uncomfortable trying to state what is right and what is wrong because they know they are not perfect, either. Often these right or wrong discussions dwindle down to,

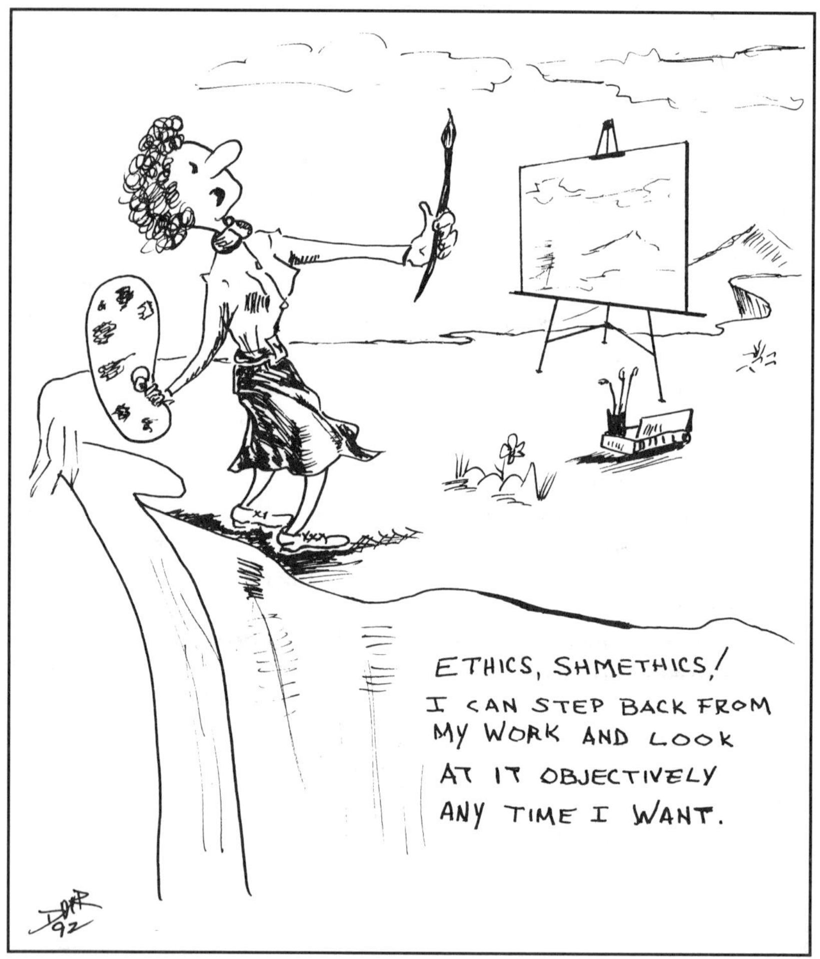

"Well, everybody is entitled to their own opinion," and usually end with, "It depends on the situation anyway."

Ivan Hill (1980) of the Ethics Resource Center at Georgetown University in Washington, DC, tells the following story related to him by a "situational ethicist":

> A pioneer woman, alone in a distant cabin with nine children, one a crying baby in her arms, heard the yells of "wild" Indians as they came toward her cabin. She took the children up to a hidden attic. Just as the Indians reached the door to the cabin, the baby cried. She smothered the baby and saved herself and the other eight children. (p. 10)

Thus, according to the situational ethicist, the situation often justifies the action—in this instance, murder. To counter, Hill poses that the situation is rather unusual, and suggests that there could be an exception even to exceptional situations. Those Indians, he offers, might have been *good* Indians, whose land and neighbors had not yet been ravaged. A person, then, should not use a one-in-a-million situation to justify release from the 999,999 obligations that remain.

In the professions, and audiology is not an exception, one needs a highly developed sense of values to reach decisions on what is ethically right or wrong. Every profession must guard against the stream of entreaties to compromise on principles. Once compromise becomes an all too easy an adjustment, one loses the backbone of conviction that allows one to make ethical decisions from the sheer habit of being ethical.

As plausible as all that may be, the uneasiness over ethics statements that proscribe a professional's relationship with product line suppliers seems to be emanating mostly from the profession of audiology. Physicians have accepted AMA ruling, pharmacists have accepted the ASHP ruling, but audiologists voice their distaste for such rigid control. The reasons they give are not always good. They seem to want it both ways, that is, to be an entrepreneur who can take uncontrolled advantage of also being a professional. They're asking for a balance, and they want to be the fulcrum. Balance may be an impossibility for some, but it also may be worth a try by everybody, at least until society in general decides what it wants in the way of health care and the calibre of health care professionals it is willing to tolerate.

ASSUMPTIONS FOR BALANCE

Some assumptions are necessary, however, in order to proceed toward developing an acceptable balance of sorts between the business of a practice and the profession of audiology. The assumptions for discussions of balance between the two are:

1. Audiologists wish to continue being identified as professionals and not entrepreneurs.
2. Consumers must be able to distinguish between audiologists (professionals) and purveyors of hearing aids (salespeople).
3. Benefits accrue to the profession when its members openly support standards of conduct that maximize the services obtained from those entrusted with their care.
4. Society is undergoing a change in what it will accept in the provision of health care, and until society arrives at a firm position, an attitude of tolerance between the ethics of professions and businesses is necessary, but the professions must be the focal point and the dominant partner.

On the belief that those assumptions are correct and are important to development of equilibrium between the professional and business ethics of the practice of audiology, a look at the need for balance may be the logical next step.

NEED FOR BALANCE

In the fall issue of *Audiology Today* Earl Harford (1991) put the concern for professionalism a slightly different way. The point is beautifully made in the guidance for establishing an independent private practice, when Harford indicates that one must decide whether to operate as a seller of hearing aids who just happens to be an audiologist, or as a professional audiologist who provides (sells) hearing aids as one phase of a comprehensive hearing health care service. There are behavioral rules that will be followed for either choice, of course, but rules are quite different for each.

If the choice is to operate as a seller of hearing aids who just happens to be an audiologist, the chances are that the Golden Rule will suffice as a guide to fair and just business practices. There is nothing wrong with that selection. Audiologists who function in that manner are not necessarily bad guys. Most perform a justifiable, respectable, and certainly not uncommon attitude of practice. Aside from the fact that the consumer of services is unable to determine whether the practitioner is a seller of hearing aids who happens to be an audiologist, or the other way around, there is an additional different and difficult slant to a predominant "sales attitude" when viewed from the position of professional associations.

The difficulty is not with the choice of operating as a seller of hearing aids who happens also to be an audiologist. The difficulty arises because one can't just "happen to be an audiologist." The status of audiologist is defined by academic preparation, clinical credential, membership in a professional association requiring certain standards of conduct, and in most states licensing that defines a scope of practice. Strictly speaking, either one is or one isn't an audiologist. There is no such thing as just happening to be an audiologist. If one qualifies as an audiologist, then one is obligated to assume the territory that goes with being a professional. The system of ethics becomes more stringent for professionals; the Golden Rule is no longer solely sufficient.

What Harford (1991) is referring to, of course, is an attitude, a mind-set, a demeanor. He is correct to point out that a seller of hearing aids is just that—a seller of hearing aids. The person could be a seller of baby picture albums, investments, automobiles, packaged meats, or shoes. The person could sell baby albums one day, automobiles the next, hearing aids the third, and on the fourth day begin the rotation all over. Nothing, except common sense, could cause that not to happen if the seller of goods desired it. The *interest* is to sell goods because the sale of goods makes money.

The seller could be something else, though, such as a world class concert pianist *and* one who sells baby picture albums, a magician who sells investments, an artist who is an auto salesperson, or an audiologist who sells hearing aids. What is common to them all is the sale of products. The obvious force driving that commonality is self-interest. The artist who sells a high number of automobiles is thought of as a good salesman not because of fine art skills, but because a great number of cars are sold. The person is not a fine artist because of a high auto sales volume, either.

The fact that such people, in addition to being salespersons, are also something else is only important in the case of the hearing aid salesperson who is an audiologist. The concert pianist who sells baby picture albums is not helped in the sale of that product because the individual is a concert pianist. The seller of hearing aids who is an audiologist, however, may very well be a more successful seller of hearing aids because of the status of being educated, credentialed, and licensed as an audiologist. The audiologist is a professional and as such commands the public trust and is obligated to preserve it. The consumer traditionally believes that a recommendation, *any* recommendation, offered by a professional is in the best interest of the consumer—and not merely the self-interest of the seller.

As a professional one cannot just "do unto others," or just do the "right thing." One has an obligation as a member of a profession to "do what is right," to assure that "the welfare of the recipient of professional services is paramount," that "self-interest" is not the motivating force shaping the services and/or products recommended for use.

An audiologist cannot be a seller of hearing aids who just happens to be an audiologist. Audiologists should not accept the cloak of respectability on the one hand by indicating that they chose the field of audiology to help people, and on the other admit that they must maintain a "perk" relationship with suppliers of merchandise to provide for the welfare of the consumer.

Unfortunately, there is grumbling among audiologists who believe they deserve the trust of their professional associations and that there is no need for an ethics standard or a policy statement to minimize their personal benefits through participation in product sales. But that plea, at least in today's marketplace, ignores what has befallen the AMA as a result of the physician nonchalance with the gift practices of the pharmaceutical houses, as one example. Other examples include restrictions placed on professionals in the military, the government, and even the limitations placed on workers employed by pharmaceutical manufacturers, themselves. All have taken refuge in a policy statement publicly making their attempt to control any negative commercial influence on the professions, that is, the appearance of impropriety.

From guidelines approved by the American Society of Hospital Pharmacists'(ASHP) Board of Directors (1991) and developed by the ASHP Council on Legal and Public Affairs[1] the following excerpts illustrate the point:

> In the practice of their profession pharmacists should be guided only by the consideration of patient care. Pharmacists should neither accept nor retain anything of value that has the potential to materially affect the ability to exercise judgments solely in the interests of patients.

The guidelines offer additional assistance to pharmacists in their relationships with industry:

> Gifts, hospitality, or subsidies offered to pharmacists by industry should not be accepted if acceptance might influence, or appear to others to influence the objectivity of clinical judgment or drug product selection and procurement.

And further,

> Pharmacists who participate in practice-based research of pharmaceuticals, devices, or other programs should conduct their activities

---

[1] The language used was adapted from documents of the American Medical Association (1991) and the American College of Physicians (1990).

in accord with basic precepts of scientific methodology. Practice-based drug studies that are, in effect, promotional schemes to entice the use of a product or program are unacceptable.

Finally,

> To avoid conflicts of interest or appearances of impropriety, pharmacists should disclose consultant or speaker arrangements or substantial personal financial holdings with companies under consideration for formulary inclusion or related decisions. To fully inform audiences, speakers and authors should disclose, when pertinent, consultant or speaker and research funding arrangements with companies.

This kind of policy statement was obviously felt necessary by the ASHP because most professionals today are subjected to powerful economic incentives taking health care professions into more of a business mode than ever before. It is a concern that might be justifiably shared by the fields of audiology and speech-language pathology.

The need for balance equally recognizes that to shut down the relationship between business and professional practice would be equally bad. Industry makes significant contributions to the growth and development of professions through financial support of educational pursuits, seminars, conferences, research funding, and so on. As much as industry relies on the professions to move product to the consumer, the professions rely on industry to aid in the development of their specialties. There is mutual benefit.

Somewhere in between the push toward commercialism emanating from the economics of modern America, and the resistance to professional links with business originating mainly, although not exclusively, from the AMA, professionals try to preserve the *professions* by appealing to their membership for self-control. In this regard it is perhaps wisest to recognize that society changes and to understand that some changes must be resisted, but some cautions must be heeded. It is perhaps *not* wise to plunge headlong into change in any profession. The AMA's caution is a reasoned position based in the tradition of an old and learned profession and driven by evidence that the pressures of commerce placed on the professions today are far greater than need be.

The caution applies to the profession of audiology, too. Audiology has barely been weaned as an independent profession. It is only just now required to fend for itself in the marketplace. While the dust is still settling audiology is looking around to see what other professions are undertaking to protect their professional image. The fork in the road looms ahead. One way leads to the preservation of a profession; the other leads elsewhere. There may be problems to face on each road.

THE PROBLEMS

The AMA asks physicians to recognize the dichotomy between professionalism and business in medical practice, and to do it in a way that will allow medicine to enter the 21st century intact as a profession. That is a necessary request, but it is one heavy with problems of the marketplace of the 90s, the cost-containment efforts of health care regulators, society's shifting values, and the moral as well as legal obligations of professions.

The issue simply put is the coexistence of two components important to the success of any professional practice—business judgments and professional ethics. There are many pieces to the puzzle in fitting these components together. At the extreme low end of the business judgments continuum are the dollar-oriented workers, where ethics frequently fly out the window. Professionals cannot remain in practice for long if they reach that extreme. At the uppermost end of the professional ethics scale are the altruistic missionaries of baseball, motherhood, and apple pie, where potentially profitable businesses, such as private practices, often die young.

It is reasonable to presume that *good* business practices are normally distributed within any group of businessmen, and similarly, to expect a bell-shaped curve of *ethical* professionals in any given profession. The concern, however, is whether the distribution will continue as normal if professional practices become predominantly businesses and the atmosphere becomes more comfortable for professional ethics to give way to self-interest.

Data released by the state of Florida Health Care Cost Containment Board indicate that in 1991 more than 40% of Florida physicians have financial interests in health care programs to which they refer patients (Issues and Facts, 1992). In an attempt to control medical costs, the federal government's Department of Health and Human Services (1992) has released the so-called "safe harbor"[2] regulations that specify acceptable investments and business arrangements for medical professionals.

Health insurance underwriters also have a vested interest in controlling health care costs. Because physicians, to a large extent, are directly responsible for the billings that health insurance eventually pays, it is not surprising that insurance carriers try to make physi-

---

[2] Issued by the U.S. Department of Health and Human Services these regulations define 11 categories protected from prosecution under the Fraud and Abuse statute (42 U. S. C. ¶ 1320a–7b). Since first enacted in 1972, Medicare/Medicaid antikickback laws have evolved to prohibit many common business arrangements for the professions.

cians be the gatekeepers of medical costs. The government has also joined the move through the Diagnosis Related Group (DRG) program which limits hospital stays by medical diagnosis. Many physicians don't like DRG because it places costs of care ahead of the welfare of the patient in some cases.

Commitment to ethics can and does mitigate the conflicts of interest inherent in any professional practice, but does not eliminate them. The salaried practitioner is not free of this problem. If financial incentives for the professional are reduced, other motives, including prestige, professional advancement, self-indulgence, family obligations, and so forth, can conflict with the care owed a patient. These can be just as detrimental to the consumer's well-being as to the practitioners's self-interest.

COST CONTAINMENT

While there will always be some irreducible quantum of self-interest in the professions, rarely, if ever, has self-interest been societally sanctioned, morally legitimized, or encouraged among the practicing professions as it is in the rationing approach to cost containment in health care. Today, for example, the physician's self-interest is deliberately used to contain the availability, accessibility, and even the quality of services to the patient. Consumers may one day just throw up their hands and cry foul.

The unavoidable situation is that the physician is in the position as primary gatekeeper for health costs (Hillman, 1989). When ethically performed, the role entails no conflict with the patients' good. Ethics and economics, individual and social good, and the physician's and patient's interests are all in congruence. As Pellegrino (1988) indicates, properly conceived and practiced medicine solves the dilemma posed in Plato's *Republic* between self-interest and the professions' altruism. It subjects the physician's art as a wage earner and as a physician to a higher standard—the standard of rational medicine, which, in turn derives its justification from being in the best interests of the patient.

NEGATIVE GATEKEEPING

Because of commercial pressures, other gatekeeping methods have crept into the arena. Each has attendant serious moral objection because the primary intent is economic, not ethical, obligation. The DRG program is one example of this "negative gatekeeping." If the number of days of hospitalization (or number of tests) assigned to a particular diagnostic group is exceeded, the hospital and/or the physician loses the differences between amount paid and costs incurred. If the number of hospitalized days (or tests) is less than the allotted amount, the institution and or physician profit. DRGs apply to hospitals who bill federally funded programs for health care hospital costs.

Another example is the preferred provider, or HMO, contract in which the practitioner or institution contracts to provide services to a prescribed number of patients for a fixed annual amount (Luft, 1978). If the total costs for care exceed the contract amount, the provider bears the loss; when costs are less, the provider profits. The essence of these plans is to motivate the provider to limit access to care by

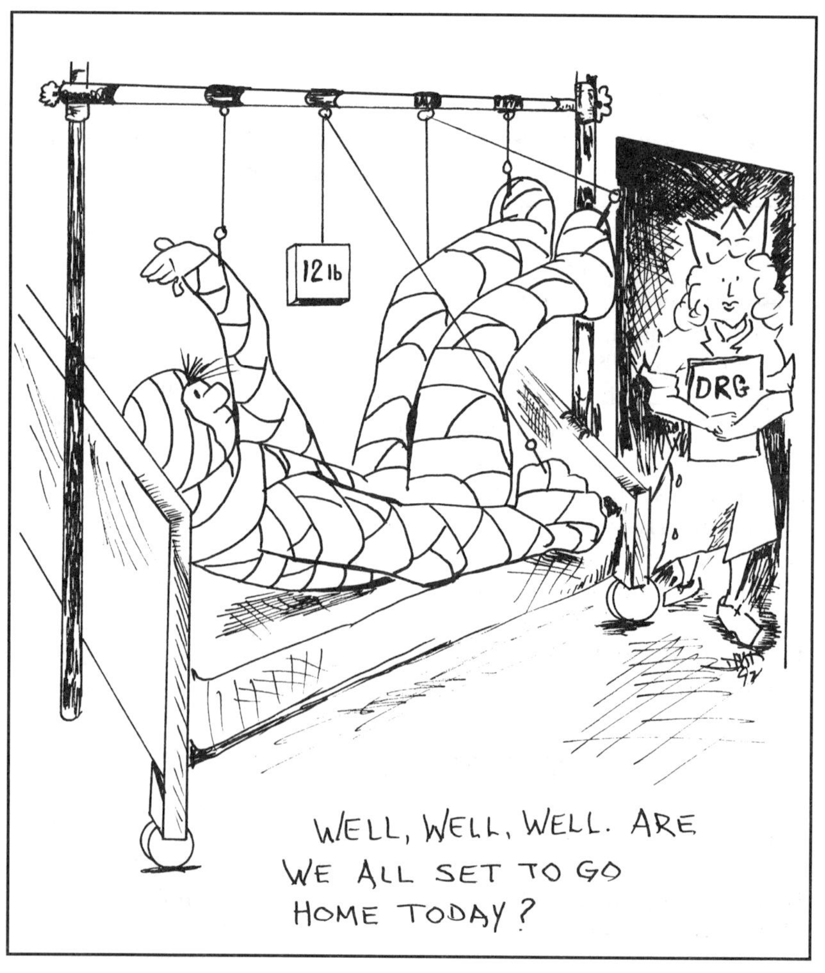

appealing to the practitioner's self-interest (Eisenberg, 1985). This is obviously an ethical dilemma.

With all these plans, the practitioner, in this case the physician, becomes the focus of incentives and disincentives. Economic efficiency is monitored and deviations from the norm are rewarded or punished. The rewards may be in the form of profit-sharing, bonuses, or promotion. The disincentives are loss of profit, limits on admitting privileges perhaps, or nonrenewal of contract (Hillman, 1987).

The major pressure, at present, is on the first contact in the system, the primary care physician who makes the majority of the decisions concerning entry into the system. Gradually, as pressures for cost containment increase, the inclusion of other practitioners as negative gatekeepers seems obvious.

POSITIVE GATEKEEPING

There is also a form of gatekeeping referred to as "positive gatekeeping." In this version the practitioner is encouraged to *increase* rather than decrease access to services. The purpose, obviously, is not to contain costs, but to enhance profits. For those who can pay, the latest and most expensive services are available. The aim is to "penetrate" and "dominate" a market and to eliminate services that are not profitable. Increasing demand for services is an implicit goal. Examples of positive gatekeeping are television commercials that advertise plastic surgery or elective surgery of all types (InterStudy Report, June 1986).

SUMMARY OF COST CONTAINMENT

Both of these forms of gatekeeping exploit the *de facto* role of the physician practitioner. Serious moral issues arise in considering the degree to which these other interests dilute the trust the patient places in the professional. The motives of self-interest on which the positive and negative aspects of gatekeeping depend complicate the irreducible quanta of self-interest that have always existed in any professional–patient relationship.

Efforts at cost containment are not, in themselves, immoral, any more than the pressures placed on professionals by industry are to be judged immoral. Both, as a matter of fact, are morally mandatory when they can be demonstrated to be in the best interest of the consumer of professional services (Siu, 1986). They violate those interests if, for whatever reason, they deny needed services, diminish the quality of services, or induce the consumer to purchase or the professional to provide unneeded services or devices.

The ethical dilemmas here, then, arise out of the manner in which economic incentives and disincentives modify the practitioner's freedom to function in the patient's behalf. The model of positive gatekeeping most closely parallels the current situation in audiology, regarding the need to balance professional and business components.

In the positive gatekeeper model the profit motive is primary. The transaction between doctor and patient is a commodity transaction—a facelift, tummy-tuck, blepharoplasty, and so on. The physician becomes an independent entrepreneur or the agent of investors who themselves have no connection with, or appreciation for, the traditions of medical ethics. The physician begins to practice the ethics of the marketplace, to interpret any relationship with the patient not as a covenant or as trust, but as a business or contract relationship. Ethics becomes, not a matter of obligations or virtue, but a matter of legality. The metaphors of business and law replace those of ethics. As generally no third party pays for hearing aids, the commodity is to be sold to those who can pay. Marketing helps, selling one's self helps, being part of a profession helps.

The positive gatekeeping model has no defensible moral argument. Ultimately it sets up a conflict between profit and patient welfare. When such a conflict occurs, it is patient welfare that suffers. There are ethicists who might say that there can be no compromises: Neither the professions nor the public can have it both ways. Either the professional primarily serves the interests of those who buy services, or the professional becomes the instrument of social and fiscal policy (Government Accounting Office, 1988).

No one knows how that will turn out, but it is fairly certain that the decision will be made by society—assuming that the American public is ready and willing to resolve the ethics dilemmas and prepared to accept the ethical conflicts of divided loyalty. Intuition and custom indicate that society may not be yet ready to abandon its moral expectation that professionals act in the patients' best interest. To some extent this is reflected by litigation in which patients hold physicians liable for harm done by discharging them too soon from the hospital, omitting tests, or even failing to hospitalize them. Because traditional expectations appear to continue the need for, at least, a balanced relationship between profession and business interest is virtually mandatory at the present time.

It may well prove correct that no one can serve two masters, no professional can be expected to balance a relationship between profession and industry, and that the great forces of cost containment will result in sweeping changes in the policy statements of the professions. Society may be willing to settle for something less than it is now enjoying in health care provision. Perhaps ethicists, moralists,

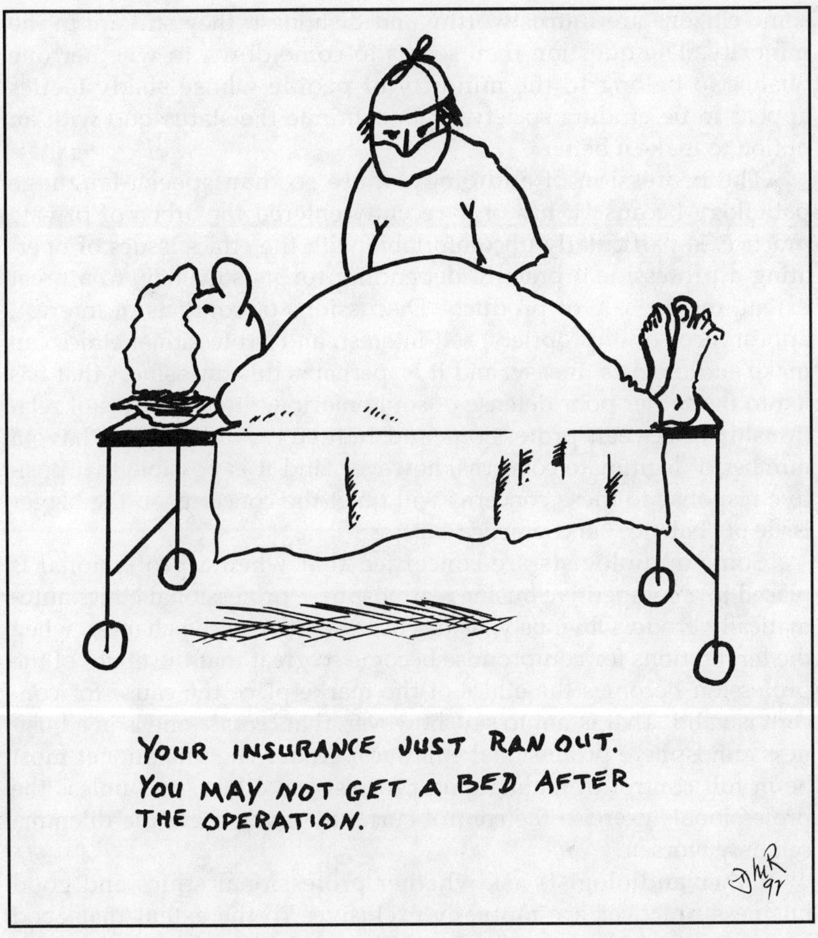

philosophers, religious leaders, industrial heads, and professionals will deliberate these issues well into the next century, but society will make the ultimate choice. Until it does the problems will not go away, and the professions remain obligated to protect the public trust in the best way possible for now.

SOME CONSIDERATIONS FOR AUDIOLOGY AND SPEECH-LANGUAGE PATHOLOGY

Most people continue throughout their lives to be honest and ethical. Hundreds and hundreds of business transactions are made daily, strictly on the basis of honesty and ethical responsibility. Although some citizens are untrustworthy and dishonest, they still are in the minority. The question then seems to come down to whether one wishes to belong to the minority of people whose shady tactics appear to be eroding society, or to continue the status quo with an option to make it better?

The profession of audiology, more so than speech-language pathology because it has only recently entered the arena of private practice, is particularly uncomfortable with the ethics issues of operating a professional practice depending for its solvency, to a great extent, on the sale of products. Discussions of conflicts of interest, appearances of impropriety, self-interest, and professional ethics can make audiologists uneasy, and it is, perhaps, this uneasiness that has led to the rather poor defense of sophomoric written controls of relationships between professions and industry. Audiologists have a number of legitimate concerns, however, and it is possible that positive response to these concerns will quiet the concerns on the bigger issue of "balance" and practice success.

Some audiologists are concerned that when a professional is placed in a competitive business atmosphere professional ethics automatically erode. Obviously, as discussed earlier in the chapter, when the temptations for compromise become so great that the ethics of the profession becomes the ethics of the marketplace the cause for concern is valid. That is not to say, however, that *because* one is in a business atmosphere professional ethics *will* erode. The practitioner must be in full control of maintaining professional ethics, and unless the professionals exercise the control currently given them the dilemma can only worsen.

Other audiologists ask whether professional ethics and good business practices are mutually exclusive. To the extent that good business practices are totally shaped by self-interest and professional practices are based in the good of the patient, the two are mutually exclusive. However, because of the way today's health care is provided and because of the dependency between professions and industry, as well as the number of technological advances in almost all health care endeavors, industries and the professions must seek equitable relationships that allow both to function and grow.

Professionals want also to know whether a private practitioner is more likely to violate a professional code of ethics than is a staff member of an institution. The individual temptations to which a private practitioner is exposed are probably greater than those proffered to a member of a program staff. Also, up to a point, a staff member of a program will probably receive a paycheck regardless of the number of services provided. A private practitioner, however, is fully reliant on the number of services provided or products sold to ensure personal income. Although the environments are different and the degrees of risk are not alike, professional practitioners who are trained in ethical practices show no more proclivity to violate an ethics code in one place or the other.

The big question for everyone, however, is whether a balance can be achieved between compliance with a code of professional ethics and the profit demands of a successful practice? The answer, of course, is yes—as long as the professional maintains control, the good of the patient is kept in the foreground, and everyone understands that it is a "balance of sorts"—a benevolent dictatorship.

SOME EXAMPLES OF CONCERNS

The answers to practitioner concerns are never easy. Although ethics monitors appreciate the concerns, they are reluctant to offer universal solutions. For example, examine the following situations and determine in your own mind whether the answers are defensible and in what circumstances they answer might not apply:

A.   In general, if an audiologist fits every corner-audiogram patient with at least one Dolce Vita ABC hearing aid, is this unethical according to the AAA code? Not necessarily, but there are instances where it might be.

B.   Are speech and hearing program staff apt to be considered in violation of the Code of Ethics of the AAA, or ASHA, merely because they have used the same earmold lab for several years? Not for that reason alone.

C.   Must an audiologist ignore all of the hearing aid discount purchase packages available in order to avoid being reported as unethical and found in violation of the AAA Code? Recall that optometrists are prohibited by their code from participating in rebate programs. There is no such clear prohibition in the Codes of Ethics governing the practice of audiology. The audiologist may be **reported**, but may not be found in violation of the code simply for taking advantage of discount purchase plans. Other transgressions associated with the discount purchase may be involved, however, which when taken into consideration would paint a different picture. Medicaid, in at least one state, is investigating the procedures used in hearing aid dispensing practices that take advantage of a manufacturer's quantity discount hearing aid purchases, but fail to reflect any savings to the reimburser, in this case the state government.

D.   Is it possible for audiologists to utilize the services of a single hearing aid manufacturer exclusively and still remain in compliance with the Academy's Code of Ethics? Probably. Unless it can be shown that a clear conflict of interest exists by doing so, that is, for example, that recipients of amplification are being misled or deceived or are receiving harmful service and so on.

E. Are speech-language pathologists who are not familiar with tracheo-esophageal puncture and the availability of the Blom-Singer prosthesis as an option for speech after laryngectomy risking non-compliance with a code of ethics that stipulates quality of service and the need for referral to other specialists? Probably not, although the safest approach is to discuss the option with patients, offering them the choice of seeking therapy elsewhere.

These examples are not testimonials, nor are they meant to serve as comprehensive models for the specific situations cited in each or as fixed interpretations of a code of ethics. They are, however, meant to illustrate the latitude extant in codes of professional conduct.

Obviously, no professional association should be so rigid and inflexible through its Code of Ethics that it is insensitive to the practice needs of its members. Neither should it be pressured into change that is motivated by other than professional ethics interests.

REMEMBER WHEN

About four decades ago, the Audivox Company produced an unique hearing aid receiver designated as the 9C. It was developed to serve individuals with normal hearing through about 2KHz and was used with an Audivox bodyaid. The size of the receiver, slightly larger than a pencil eraser, was revolutionary for those days. Most importantly it achieved unmatched success in fitting the young hearing-impaired military population with a high percentage of precipitous, high frequency hearing loss from war noise exposure.

Audiologists serving the military population quickly came to rely on the benefits of the Audivox 9C receiver and some utilized it to the *exclusion* of other available purported "high frequency emphasis" hearing aids. Although the matter of professional ethics was not as talked about then as now, no one was reported for overuse of a specific item from a sole manufacturing source. There was never a question that pressure was being exerted by the manufacturer or that a huge rebate to the government was being passed out. The question of ethics was never raised. Of course, audiologists were not selling these hearing aids.

Audiologists in private practice become acquainted with suppliers of product and tend to favor some over others for a variety of legitimate reasons. Professional ethics would dictate that this type of favoritism be driven by the need to provide the *best* for a patient, and not be motivated by an eagerness to accumulate "buyer" points for conversioned into a future ticket to Shangri-la. When a professional puts self-interests ahead of all else, professional ethics are put at risk.

TO TELL OR NOT TO TELL

Consider a hypothetical situation involving a dentist who, early in practice, located a dental supply company that in the practitioner's opinion made outstanding filling material. The dentist has, in fact, purchased all filling material from this company for nearly 15 years. The order to the company has consistently requested 50 pounds every month, except for a few times over the years when the order dropped below 50 pounds because the dentist went on a long vacation. But the supplier considers the dentist a regular 50-pound-per-month buyer.

One day a sales rep from the company called on the dentist and said, "Doctor, if you buy 75 pounds of this **new** amalgam each month for the next 12 months, not only will I give it to you cheaper by the pound than you're now getting it, but I will install a Jacuzzi in your bathroom. I'll leave this brochure. It describes the new amalgam and our purchasing program—you know, all about how you get the Jacuzzi and even some other things."

The dentist has a decision to make at this point. The approach selected can affect both the business and the professional aspects of the practice. The decision will also describe whether the dentist is driven by professionalism or self-interest.

The dentist could say, "Terrific! I've always wanted a Jacuzzi in my bathroom and I know they're not cheap. I'm sure I can fill a few more cavities a week to use the extra amalgam. I usually let the little ones go for a time. I'll just fill 'em sooner that's all. It won't make any difference to the patient."

Conversely, the rep could be told, "Fine, but I don't want the Jacuzzi, so whatever you figure the cost of it is just reduce what you charge me for the filling material that much more. That way I can further increase my profit margin and put a few more dollars in the bank so I can take two months' vacation next year. Maybe three."

Or the dentist could respond, "Okay I'll take the 75 pounds of the new stuff. But, I would rather you reduce my cost for the amalgam by the cost of the Jacuzzi because I already have a Jacuzzi, and I don't want two Jacuzzis. To be honest with you I don't even want the one Jacuzzi, but my spouse thinks it's fun. Besides, I can put the savings back into the practice and perhaps not have to raise the charge to my patients for fillings next year."

Still another rejoinder might be simply to say to the sales rep, "Thanks but no thanks. Just deliver my regular 50 pounds. That's all I ever use. That's all I need. And besides I still have some left from three years ago when I went on vacation for a month, and you wouldn't take back. The old stuff works just fine for me."

At least one of these responses would be an excellent choice for the **good of the business**. It may **not** be a **professionally ethical** choice, but it would be a good business judgment. Another selection might be the **purely ethical** approach, but an **eventual disaster** to business growth and the future of the practice. One of the choices is defensible because it embodies **balance between professional and business ethics**, no detriment comes to the quality of care provided the patient, and the dentist remains in control of the offer.

In the above situations, thought must also be given to the patients of the dentist. Remember, patients have the right to expect impartiality from a professional. They do not suspect that professionals are motivated by anything other than a strong desire to provide what is *best* for them. Patients do not approach a professional person alert for what may be a conflict of interest. The patient affords the professional complete trust. That's the tradition. Professions have earned the public trust because they have not engaged in conflicts of interest.

How might the patient's attitude toward the dentist change, however, if the dentist openly displayed the company's brochure describing the Jacuzzi offer for a 12-month purchase guarantee? For one thing the patient might wonder if the dentist were filling the patient's tooth because it truly required filling, or because the dentist made more money as a result of company discounts associated with greater use of material. Or the patient might wonder if the dentist were using a lot of amalgam in order to qualify for the Jacuzzi.

Would any of the conclusions drawn from this model change if the scenario were altered to apply directly to the fields of speech-language pathology and audiology. Probably not.

A rule of thumb in situations involving product promotions might be that, if you as a professional would feel comfortable telling all your patients truthfully about the promotional arrangements you maintain with the suppliers of goods you sell, the chances are good that the arrangements are professionally ethical. But, if you are hesitant to reveal to your patients that the sale of an "x" number of Dolce Vita hearing aids, for example, results in you being flown to Shangri-la, the possibility of the arrangements being a violation of the Code of Ethics is increased significantly.

Disclosure is not a full solution to the problem, however, because it does not take into account that patients depend on the professionals' unbiased judgment to select what is best for them—whether that means a choice of treatment, or a prosthetic device. Disclosing a manufacturer's incentive rebate plan to a patient in no way renders the patient better able to judge the differences among products in the way a professional can. The patient *still* relies on the practitioner's judgment. Patients may think they are getting something when, in fact, they are not.

Frustrating as it may be, a good business decision is not always a professionally ethical one. In opposite fashion, a professionally ethical conduct may not always provide for the best business tactics. The pure business person has no professional ethic to consider when charging the corner-audiogram patient $2,400 for binaural hearing aids, for instance. There is only the ethic of the marketplace—present and future. The audiologist as a professional, however, always must be aware that self-interest is rarely a proper motivation toward compliance with a Code of Ethics. The professional, especially the private practitioner, must constantly strive to preserve an appropriate balance between the necessary ethics of professionalism and the good sense of business. The "wolf at the door" is usually not a friendly animal.

7

In Whose Interest Is It?

A long habit of not thinking a thing wrong gives it the superficial appearance of being right. (Thomas Paine)

Neil Levy (Levy & Mishkin, 1990), legal advisor to the Ethical Practices Board of the American Speech-Language-Hearing Association and a partner in the Washington, DC, law firm of Hogan and Hartson, supports the view that there is a clear and accepted distinction between the motivations that drive a salesperson and those that steer a professional. That is not to indicate that salespeople as a group fail to heed The Golden Rule or as a group have a poor moral standard. It is, however, to state what should be obvious to the professional; the ethics of a professional are justifiably expected to be at a higher level than the ethics of a nonprofessional.

Despite the likelihood that many business people would like to debate that issue, the fact of the matter is that it *is* the fact of the matter. The conflict between economic and patient interests lies close to the surface in all patient care relationships. The ethics implications of this conflict for those responsible for managing or providing health care services are enormous. Maintaining the higher level of professional ethics is becoming more and more difficult because of competitive pressures.

It is the public that health care organizations serve, and all actions must be measured against and directed toward the goal of protecting patients and furthering their interests. That is the heartbeat of a profession. When individuals elevate the interest of business and self-interest above the interests of the people served that is the heartbeat of commercialism. When self-interest assumes the dominant position, it is time for the buyer to beware.

CAVEAT EMPTOR AS IT APPLIES TO THE PROFESSIONS

As a consumer one accepts that there is a strong degree of self-interest influencing the used car salesman who says, "You can't afford to pass up this little cream puff driven by a nonsmoking little old lady to and from church. This car is meant for you, my friend, this car is meant for you!"

The salesman is there to sell cars. The more sold, the more money goes into his or her pocket. If you manage to get off the lot without consummating a sale, you get a phone call later, or a letter, stating the car is still available and maybe at a better price. Some people say "Caveat emptor! (let the buyer beware)," whenever one buys products. Levy and Mishkin (1990) ask, "In whose best interest is it anyway?"

Consider the situation that surrounds a visit to the family pediatrician. Does a mother think, "Caveat emptor," or ask, "In whose best interest is it anyway?" when the physician says the infant needs vitamin drops? Is there a concern that the doctor is acting out of self-interest, is the doctor building business for the pharmacy—or rather is there automatically the belief that the doctor has the best interest of the patient uppermost?

As an example, in the case of *Wolff v. McDonnell* (1974) a dentist informed a patient that a tooth must be extracted from the lower jaw to guard against future erosion of the mandible under the reportedly abscessed tooth. It was further recommended that the space left by the extracted tooth be filled with a bridge arrangement. The extraction cost $175 and the bridge $2,800.

Because of circumstances following the extraction and later because of an ill-fitting bridge, the patient initiated legal action against the dentist. The patient claimed that the dentist made an initial misdiagnosis resulting in the needless extraction of a tooth, later causing postextraction pain, suffering, and neuralgia, allegedly the fault of a poorly made bridge. The patient also reported the dentist to the ethics monitors of the dental association.

The point here is that the patients in both of these instances put full trust and confidence in the professional practitioners, as would be expected. As a patient one does not often question the recommendation of a professional. This is true primarily because a patient does not suspect a professional's judgments as being based in anything other than the best interest of the patient. Patient-initiated second opinions are more common than in the past, however.

When an audiologist tells a patient "This is the best hearing aid for you," the traditional patient's assumption would be that the recommendation would be influenced by the audiologist's professional and independent judgment based in a genuine expertise in selecting the best device to ameliorate the condition that led to the consultation. A consumer of professional services does not automatically wonder if self-interest is a stimulant for a professional's judgment. Caveat emptor is not a suitable caution when applied to the professions.

The buyer of services or products from a representative of a profession should not have to beware. They should be confident that the practitioner is able to render judgments free from commercial influence and the pressures of the marketplace.

SCENARIOS

As indicated in Chapter 1, the attitude of trust toward the professions, in general, may be changing because of societal shifts. Those shifts are putting great pressures on professions. The question of what happens to a professional's obligations to a consumer when practitioners are surrounded by pressures that give even the *appearance* of conflict is raised. Consumers want to know whether the established obligations are being watered down and whether they should expect less from a professional in the '90s than they did in the '60s.

Professionals want to know how to recognize the pressures, and organizations want to know how to assist their members protect the interests of the profession and ensure the protection of the consuming public without taking on the semblance of paternalism.

These questions are of major concern to ethical practice boards throughout the country. A shared belief among entities is that any action between a third party outside the professionals' association and the professional must clearly support the following principles:

A. Hold the interest of the patient/client paramount;

B. Promote and preserve the interest/image of the profession at large;

C. Conform to an objective Code of Professional Conduct enabling self-regulation by the profession when its members fail to conform to published principles.

While keeping these three principles in mind, consider the following imagined scenarios and make your own best determination of whose best interest is served in each instance:

Scenario 1: Potential Buyer Influence

In the office of the new Director of Clinical Services for a large metropolitan hospital on the West Coast, the telephone rang early one morning. The voice of a manufacturer's rep from a well-known company doing a modest business with the hospital through the Clinical Service Program says, "Good morning, Doctor! How are you today? I'll be in your town on Friday and I wonder if you can get away for a nice lunch? Or dinner, if you'd rather. Bring your spouse. It'll be a nice evening. What do you say?"

Even though it is entirely possible that the caller is truly a friendly, gregarious person, an undertone of influence peddling permeates the invitation. Of course, it is quite possible for the Director of the Clinical Services Program to accept the invitation in good faith, believing that the influence of a lunch or dinner is too minimal to be persuasive for using or overusing the product represented by the invitation.

Although not totally clear, on the surface it is likely that accepting the invitation would be judged unethical under each of the three principles specified above. What is clear is that:

1. Accepting the invitation can in no way serve a client's best interest;
2. Accepting the invitation can affect or appear to affect, the director's inclination to procure the goods of this manufacturer rather than try out others that may, in reality, be better; and
3. The interests of the profession are not served when professional conduct leads to a public impression that a gratuity is being accepted when the motive is obviously to influence the conduct of the professional.

There is a high probability of influence in the first scenario, but the ability of an ethics board to demonstrate the existence of any influence is actually quite low. The risk to consumers and the reputation of the profession should make the acceptance of such an invitation unacceptable in a strong profession. In any case, the risks outweigh any benefits that may accrue to consumers, professionals, or organizations allowing such conduct. An objective ethics code should prohibit the behavior. Most codes do not clearly stipulate such a prohibition, however.

Scenario 2: Targeted Influence

At the annual Convention of the United Academy of Osteopathy, a pharmaceutical company with a table set up in the registration area makes an outright cash gift to each academy member at the time of registration. The note on the little card accompanying the $100 bill says, "We just want you to know you are important to us."

There is no way that this imaginary example conforms to any of the guiding principles of ethics. This type of influence should be prohibited by an objectively stated code of ethics. There should be no room for allowing a practitioner's subjective belief that personal judgment would be unaffected by money. Truthfully speaking, it would be extraordinarily difficult for a board to determine whether a particular practitioner's judgment was altered by such a gift, but it is that very difficulty that demands a prohibition be based on a purely objective standard.

Drug companies, not unlike other commercial enterprises, would not give away money for nothing. What they would hope to get in return, and more often than not DO get in return, is a handle on the practitioner's judgment. The public, remember, assumes that the professional's judgments are free from allegiance to or influence from vendors of product.

Scenario 3: Captive Influence

A hearing aid manufacturer wants to call audiologists' attention to a new line of hearing aids by offering its audiologist customers an expense paid trip to Hilton Head, SC, in January for a 4-day seminar. The seminar program is consists of company officials' greetings, welcomes, farewells, and an afternoon of technical presentations on the seminar first day. The remainder of the time can be at the attendees' discretion, ranging from a calendar from a calendar of "Duffer's Golf Classic"; "Swinger's Tennis Tournament"; sail boating, scuba diving, snorkeling, fishing, drinking, dancing, and several other options, including a visit to the exhibit room.

The conventional justification for such programs is that consumers in the long run benefit from professionals, in this case audiologists, receiving the information imparted at such gatherings. Stated another way, the program is justified as serving the best interest of the product's consumer.

Recall that marketing requires getting people's attention. Certainly an expense-paid trip to a warm climate in January is an effective marketing ploy. The purported educational value of such programs is repudiated by the disproportionately small amount of the program devoted to serious teaching activity. High-minded intent is severely undercut by the obvious coincidence of the right place at the right time.

There is nothing wrong with well-written, published articles objectively explaining the company claims about a new line. An expense-paid trip is a targeted event, unlike the random giveaway that is another way of communicating, "...if you're free for lunch..." as in Scenario 1, or giving $100 to practitioners who just happened to attend the convention. The trip to Hilton Head, probably offered several times during each year's winter months, would be by invitation. Such a marketing method helps expand the influence of the vendor on a specific practitioner's judgment in the context of an ongoing commercial relationship.

The public image of the profession runs great risk of being tarnished. Most professions would be well advised to divorce themselves from situations in which a professional's judgment can even appear to be intermixed with vendor promotional activities. An objective code of ethics would prohibit such activity to the extent that it can by stating clear definitions to distinguish between genuine scientific meetings and those that are clearly vacation excursions with only a veneer of substance.

Scenario 4: Rebates

A contact lens manufacturer offers a buyers' incentive to participating optometrists: 5% off the price of each pair of lenses purchased beyond the first 100 pairs; an additional 8% off after the second 100 pairs, and 18% off all pairs purchased beyond 200.

The influence of a discount program or other kind of rebate accrual program on the patients' best interest and the interest of the profession in light of the guiding principles is certainly less clear than in the preceding examples. Yet, the obvious question persists on the effect such an incentive program has on an optometrist's judgment in choosing lenses for a patient. The glib answer is simply to say that a discount incentive would have no affect on a professional recommendation. But it might, and that's the issue.

One could question whether the potential problem would be alleviated if an optometrist would disclose such a discount program to all patients receiving contact lenses. In conjunction is the question of whether public trust in the profession would be undermined irrevocably if the details of such programs were made known to the consuming market. There are no pat answers. But, it would seem that if professions want to remain professions—and not just businesses with higher trained personnel—preservation of the founding principles and values of professions, in general, should be of paramount concern.

Obviously, profit incentives can tend to mark a profession by creating a motive for self-interest, rather than the interest of those served professionally. Where substantial likelihood exists that professionals will be influenced, or appear to be influenced, to prefer their own self-interest over that of the patient, and where the consumer *has no way of knowing the difference*, the practice should be unacceptable within a code of ethics.

Perhaps practitioners in some professions would feel comfortable disclosing purchase incentive programs to their patients. Perhaps not. Unfortunately, disclosure is not a simple cure-all. Informing a patient of such a program does not really help the patient determine if the professional is acting in the best interest of the patient. Neither does disclosure equip the patient to evaluate the choices among various health care products with the skill of a professional. A code of ethics should clarify the boundaries. These boundaries should be based on the most objective standards possible for the profession. It is not good enough to judge an incentive discount program as ethical simply because the using practitioner believes deep down that personal financial benefit is not affecting the clinical judgment on which patients rely.

Scenario 5: Quotas and Quality of Service

A provider of speech-language pathology services, "Splang, Inc.," has contracted with a nursing home. Under the contract "Splang, Inc." must require its employees to perform a minimum of 38 patient contact hours per week. One of "Splang's" employees believes this is unethical.

In this instance the question is one of quality of service. Imposing a quota conflicts with the first guiding principle, which indicates that the welfare of the patient is paramount. Imposing a quota is a step toward undercutting professionalism. That is not to suggest that the need to meet expenses needs to be sacrificed for the sake of ethics. It is to indicate that ethical antennae should be aroused when there is incentive for a professional to behave as though the product of health care service is so many widgets to be fabricated at so many per hour.

It is quite likely that the example quota imposition would be judged unethical. There are data available through the American Speech-Language-Hearing Association describing the number of cases that can be managed by a speech-language pathologist without sacrificing quality of service. These data can objectively support the deterioration in quality of individual services when quotas are set too high.

Scenario 6: Credit Where Credit is Due

The chair of the Department of Speech and Language at a university enlists the help of a doctoral student to collect and analyze records of patients in the university hospital's Closed-Head Trauma Unit (CHTU). The records review produced material judged worthy of publication.

The doctoral student drafted the article at the request of the chair, assuming credit as a coauthor. When the article appeared, the student was mentioned in a concluding "acknowledgements paragraph," but not as an author. The student reported the incident as unethical.

Although no agreement was implied at the time of the requests to collect data and draft an article, the student's assumption of being named as a coauthor was probably justified on the basis of the amount of work provided. Additionally, as stated in paragraph C of the above criteria, ASHA's code objectively specifies how situations such as this are to be handled. With the information presented here, it is likely that the action of the chair in excluding the student from authorship recognition would be determined to be unethical.

All these scenarios present a few of the many possibilities needed to develop ethical thinking. The reader is urged to ponder each at some length and to examine the ramifications of various options. Most professionals want to behave ethically and *do* conduct an ethical professional practice. Some, nevertheless, need a boost in recognizing and resolving ethical issues. These scenarios offer fairly simple cases. Most cases of possible ethics infractions are abundantly more complex, especially those that involve business judgments as well.

THE BUSINESS ETHICS SCENARIO

Laura L. Nash (1988), assistant professor of business administration at the Harvard Business School, has spent a year-and-a-half researching business and ethics. She advocates a process of self-questioning to test pragmatically the ethical content of decisions made in business settings. The following scenario invokes Nash's 12 questions (here adapted). Although the setting is a business venue, the paradigm and the questions easily apply to a private professional health care practice.

At the annual shareholders meeting of "Splang Inc.," Chairman and CEO "John Q. Moneybags" speaks to the group of investors assembled in the conference room:

> "As you all know, our responsibility to the consumer of speech and language services has always come first at Splang, and we continue to strive in every way toward serving our public in the absolute best way possible in the firm and sincere belief that good ethics is good business.... Despite our forecast of a continuing economic downtrend through 1994, I am pleased to announce that earnings per share were up again in 1991 for the sixth year in a row. Through the use of prudent business decisions we intend to do better again next year."

The address certainly suggests that the CEO of "Splang" believes corporate operations and corporate values are dynamically intertwined. But one of the shareholders in attendance is a philosopher, who stands and says:

> "Have we gathered all the facts here? That is to say, are our profits solely dependent on our workers being in contact with X number of consumers per day, and, if that is the case, would our profits be greater if the contacts were raised to X plus 2 or 3? But even before that we should know whether X is reasonable in an ethics sense."

As the philosopher goes on, a difficulty becomes apparent: Corporate executives and philosophers approach things in radically different ways. The academician ponders the intangible, salivates over the paradoxical, and embraces the peculiar. Philosophers speak in different languages—languages of categorical imperatives and deep theoretical viewpoints about ethics. Ethics lumbers along while the world of practical business concerns constantly measures a wide range of competing claims on time and resources weighed against the unrelenting pressures of the marketplace.

Another shareholder, a physician, speaks:

> "Perhaps there is a point here. I would like to ask, Mr. Chairman and Philosopher, if you have examined the situation of increased profits from the other side? In other words, can our workers continue to provide a level of service consistent with Splang's values?"

The question is a good one that will allow some calculation of self-interest. There is a power in self-examination, because it incorporates an exploration of the likely consequences of a decision taken from the viewpoint of those who do not immediately benefit, in this case the employees of "Splang, Inc.," who must work harder. Looking at the possible effects of a decision from the eyes of those who will feel the result directly may often result in discomfort. That discomfort should prompt a disinclination to choose the expedient over the most (professionally) responsible course of action. It doesn't always do that when business ethic is the single, unrelenting concern.

"Mrs. Harley Sanderson," wife of the owner of "Harley Sanderson Motors," addresses The CEO from her seated position in the front row:

> "John, how in the world did we get in this position anyway? I know we're all investors here, shareholders and all, but are we supposed to keep making more and more money every year by having our workers, the same NUMBER of workers see more and more people? Where will it stop? I mean aren't there laws or something, John?"

What only the CEO knows is that "Splang Inc." is about to have a competitor in town, "Speech Services Unlimited." The CEO anticipates losing 20% of the market over the next 18 months. Therefore, the CEO has deemed it prudent to increase the number of consumer contacts per worker. Vital in determining the ethics of the situation is the inquiry into its history. As "Mrs. Harley Sanderson" asks, "How did we get in this position?"

"Splang's" traditional emphasis has been on profit, that is, more contacts, more billings. Quality of service has deteriorated and, although contacts have increased, this is because consumers are seen sometimes twice a day; it is not the result of an increase in consumer base. The very decision that the CEO was about to make would probably exacerbate the situation. A look into the past is often beneficial in setting a professionally ethical future course.

In determining the ethics of the situation it is important to separate the symptoms from the disease. More of the same is not always the best solution. The question of how one got into a given mess is an important phase of self-examination.

Also important, for the CEO in this case, or for a professional in a practice setting, is to ask to what and to whom does one give personal loyalties in a corporation (practice)? To one's practice? Supervisor? Family? Society? Self? Color? Sex? It is helpful to role play a little by asking, for example, "How might I respond if my daughter asks me why I did that?" If the answer is, "Because that's the way the world functions," then your loyalties are clear, and moral passivity is inevitable. But if the question causes you real problems, you probably have started to enhance your professional responsibility by asking some tough questions.

Seventy-nine-year-old Bob Gender stands with the aid of a gold cane grip to speak: "What is your intention in making this decision, Johnnie? And how does whatever your intention might be compare with the likely results? Have you thought about that?"

These two questions are tough. If the CEO had first asked them of himself it might have aided him in alleviating the reality between the disparities of intent and result. Intents *do* matter. "Splang's" motives, whether purely for profit or purely for altruism, will have wide-reaching effects inside and outside the corporation—on attitudes toward the corporation, on wages, on services of the workers, on overall attitudes toward the field of the workers training, on other investors, on other like corporations. Sociologist Max Weber (Nash, 1988) refers to this as an "ethics of attitude" and contrasts it with an "ethics of absolute ends."

An ethics of attitude sets a standard to ensure a certain action. Sound familiar? To explain the ethics of result requires a jump to the future in the scenario and the added assumption that Moneybags got his way and increased the workers' contact per day quota. Briefly looking into the future, then, it is seen that 10 months after the shareholders meeting everything went sour at "Splang," and Moneybags wishes he had never done what he did. The workers are leaving and new ones don't want to work as hard; letters have been received from the state commerce licensing board and the licensing board for the workers; a letter has come from the ethics committee of the association the workers belong to—no one is benefiting from "Splang" services, and worst of all, "Speech Services Unlimited" decided not to enter the area.

The goodness of intent pales before results that perpetrate harm, or simply do little good. "John Q. Moneybags" may have learned that knowledge of the future is most often inadequate and that overconfidence often precedes a grievous mistake. But enough of the future. Back to the current shareholders meeting as someone else asks: "Could your intention to boost profits hurt anyone?"

That question presses the point of whether potential injury is intentional or not. It is one that automobile makers ask when electing not to include certain safety measures on new car models. Given the limits of knowledge, yet aware that "Splang" ministers to sick people, the question probes for moral justification. To settle this issue at the outset is not common, but to do so would reshape the way modern corporations examine their own morality. Businesses often formulate policies on injury only after the fact. Witness, for example, the Alaskan oil spills or the Chernoble nuclear disaster.

"Could we have a discussion with the workers and anyone else who may be affected by your actions before you reach a decision, 'John?'" asks a lady in the third row.

Another excellent question asking for something that most CEOs often reject. The participation of affected parties is one of the best means of gaining information about the possible consequences of a business decision. Consider, for instance, the case of a corporate foundation that constructs a tennis court for disadvantaged youngsters in a neighborhood where most children suffer from chronic malnutrition. What a waste of resources!

The philosopher again: "Are you confident that your decision will be as valid in 2 years as it seems to you now? Given the exigencies of the marketplace and the . . . blah, blah, blah."

As anyone knows who has had to consider long-range plans and short-term budgets at the same time, a difference in time frame can change the consequences of an action. The ethical flavor of a business decision is no exception.

"Drew Conover," editor of a weekly newspaper published in a bedroom community of the city where "Splang" does most of its business, has been taking notes of the shareholder proceedings. He stands, summarizes briefly, and reads a question from his yellow pad:

> "As I understand it, you have found, in your opinion, sufficient reason to adjust—that is, increase—the company's productivity in the future, especially in the next year. At least you predict Splang, and therefore the investors, will do even better next year. My question is: Could you disclose your plans—that is, your decision—without reservation to all of us—the workers and society as a whole? Because this is a privately owned company and I am here at the invitation of your public relations director, how are you going to react when I run your plans as a headlined story in the newspaper?"

A business may maintain that there's really no problem, but there may be a number of trivial actions it is reluctant to discuss. Disclosure is a means of sounding those submarine depths of conscience.

"John Q. Moneybags," Chairman and CEO of "Splang Inc.," rises to the question of publication and the apparent risk of other reporters delving into the business of "Splang":

> "Well no, Drew, I wouldn't object to disclosing all of this and to having your paper run a story about what we're doing here. But you should also publish that we are making a sizable financial contribution to the Happy Nest Nursing Home and the City Hospital's Cochlear Implant Fund. And in the parking lot of the building here we're going to erect a backboard so the kids in the area can shoot some baskets. We have some money to do that and that's what we plan to do."

Drew Conover, still standing with his yellow pad goes on:

> "Well, there's certainly a symbolic value to that gesture, John. I hope it's understood by the community. But what if it's misunderstood?"

If the symbolic gesture is understood as the CEO of "Splang" intends, the gift may stave off any future disaffection from employees or the community, or, for that matter, consumers of "Splang's" services. It may also signal the community that "Splang" places a premium on community relations. If the symbolic value of the gesture is misunderstood, however, or if the newspapers just happen to uncover previously unknown "Splang, Inc." dealings connected to the profits of previous years and makes the business a target of the local press, the donations could then be interpreted as little more than an effort to pay off the community to ignore the company's negative aspects.

The point is that a business decision has a symbolic value of sending a signal about what is acceptable behavior in the corporate culture. How the symbol is actually perceived or misperceived is as important as it is intended to be understood.

The meeting of the shareholders drones on. What has become apparent is that the CEO had not anticipated the concerns of the investors or the exploration of the effect of his decisions on the workers, the community, the consumer, and others. The values and the consistency of the corporation are under investigation by the shareholders. There is a strong hint that some concern for maintenance of professional values looms. A final question comes from the philosopher:

> "John, if you would increase the work efforts of the staff generating revenue, would you also increase the work time of the secretarial and other support staff? If you would do X, would you as well do Y, and what might they expect as inducement?"

Every business decision has an important symbolic value. The need for consistency is obvious. It is also important to know under which conditions the rules of the game might be changed. What conflicting principles, circumstances, or constraints would set a morally acceptable basis for making an exception to one's normal business (professional) ethic?

Posing questions on consistency offers a means of eliciting the ethics of a business or of oneself. Such queries effectively test the strength, idealism, or practicality of those business or personal values. The questions also provide an adaptable means of probing what midground might be reached on the ethics of the profession a business is attempting to embrace.

"Splang," for example, had for the past 5 years sent holiday gifts to institutions with which it had maintained a contractual relationship. The shareholders' questions prompted an in-depth self-examination of the business and "Splang" looked into its policy of holiday giving. What was the acceptable limit for a gift—a bottle of scotch whiskey? A case? Does it matter that "Splang" never *intends* the gifts to be inducements? Does the possibility of inducement taint the gift? Was the cutoff limit absolute? "Moneybags" couldn't agree on a point for allowing some gifts and not others. So, a new policy was circulated, prohibiting the business from offering gifts and stating as inappropriate for its employees to receive any. The 12 questions for examining the ethics of a business/professional decision (Nash, 1988) as adapted are:

1. Is the problem accurately defined?
2. Would the definition of the problem change if it were looked at from another perspective?

3. What is the history leading to the problem?
4. To whom do you give your loyalties as a business person and as a professional?
5. Is your intention in solving the problem to improve values?
6. What are the probable results of solving the problem and how do they fit your intentions?
7. Could your solution to the problem be injurious to anyone?
8. Could you discuss the problem and the solution with the affected parties?
9. Will your solution be valid in the future?
10. Could you go public with your decision?
11. Is there a symbolic intent to your decision and what are the consequences if it is misunderstood?
12. Would you allow exceptions to your decision and under what circumstances?

The 12 main questions asked by the shareholders provided a means to articulate the responsibilities involved and to expose each for evaluation. According to Nash (1988) there are compelling reasons for holding discussions of this type:

A. The process facilitates group discussion of a topic that has, by tradition, been reserved for the privacy of one's conscience. For those whose consciences twitch a little but don't talk to them in complete sentences the questions help them to understand their own perceptions of a problem.
B. The process aids in building a cohesiveness as points of consensus emerge and people from different backgrounds become aware that they share common concerns.
C. It acts as an information resource.
D. It helps expose ethical inconsistencies in the expressed, or implied values of the business (practice).
E. Sometimes it helps to uncover differences between values and the practicality of implementing them.
F. It reveals how those involved with the business may be drawing on the private self to enhance business activity or even the reverse.
G. By drawing out self and exploring the corporation's activities, the process aids in deriving meaning from an environment that is often thought of as meaningless.
H. It helps to improve the extent and range of alternatives
I. The process is cathartic.

Another encompassing virtue of the questioning process is that it limits the level of inquiry. For example, the 12 questions explore what harm might come from a particular decision and what good is intended, but they do not probe the meaning of "good" or whether the result is "just." Philosophizing is held to a minimum. The questions do, nonetheless, presume some difference between corporate goodness and private goodness—a crucial distinction in ethics inquiry.

WHAT IS EXPECTED OF AN ETHICAL PRACTICE?

Professional practitioners, much like corporate executives, want to know what is expected of the ethical practice. Is a practice considered ethical merely because it obeys some standards of behavior, some perhaps based in archaic tradition and some considered as good principles? Here are three examples of "goodness" representing prevailing social opinions:

1.   The most rigid moral analogy to the good, or fully ethical, practice would be the "good person," as in "You're a good kid, Charlie Brown." An abstract, philosophical ideal having highly moral connotations, the "good person" label embodies an intricate relation to a number of other abstractions such as courage, godliness, righteousness, and even prudence. The achievement of this type of "good," or ethical, practice, implies a heavy responsibility to know the rules of achieving what is good and to have the *resolution* and *fortitude* to achieve it.

2.   There is also the purely amoral definition of good, as, for example, in "a good pizza"—a fulfillment (without moral judgment) of a largely inanimate and functional purpose—that is, a judgment of goodness with no consideration of whether the pizza was made from stolen dough or baked by escaped convicts. Under this definition, practice goodness would be reached by the unadorned accrual of profits with no regard for the social implications of the means of accruing profits.

3.   Somewhere between these two extremes lies the view of good as in "good dog." In this concept, goodness is achieved from the fulfillment of a social contract based on avoiding social injury. Moral capacity is present alright, but its potential is limited. One can make a moral evaluation of the good dog, but it exists primarily in concrete terms. For instance, one does not have to identify the dog's intentions as utilitarian to agree that its ethical fulfillment of the social contract is reached when it does not soil the carpet or eat the baby.

Business ethics operate most appropriately when attempting to explore and define the morality of the business at the level of the good doggie. The good business is expected to avoid dumping irretrievable harm on society while focusing on its purposes as a profit-generating venture. The moral capacity of a business, however, does not extend to determining by itself what will generally improve the overall social welfare.

The "good dog" theory of inquiry operates in concrete experience. As the 12 questions posed by the shareholders in the last scenario set a limit to moral expectations, so, too, do they place a limit on the use of abstraction to get at the problem. The model does not fit glove-like to the situations that confront the ethics of professions, but it's a beginning.

Professions operate from a different base, one some ethicists feel is mutually exclusive of the corporate ethic, if for no other reason than that business is profit driven and all commercial problems are solved with only that in mind. In the final analysis, that may turn out to be confirmed. But by avoiding theoretical inquiry and limiting expectations of goodness to a few rules for social behavior based on common sense it may be possible to develop a conduct acceptable to the professions and appropriate to the ethics, language, ideology, and institutional dynamics of a professional practice. It might even be in everybody's best interest.

The moral embraced by the following story may provide a valued lesson.

The Rabbit and the Goat[1]

A Goat once approached a peanut stand that was kept by a Rabbit, purchased five cents worth of peanuts, laid down a dime, and received a punched nickel in change. In a few days the Goat came back, called for another pint of peanuts, and offered the same nickel in payment; but in the meantime had plugged the hole in it with a peg.

"I can't take that nickel," said the Rabbit.

"This is the very nickel you gave me in change a few days ago," replied the Goat.

"I know it is," continued the Rabbit, "but I made no attempt to deceive you about it. When you took the coin the punched hole was wide open, and you could see it for yourself. In working that mutilated coin off on you I simply showed my business sagacity; but now you bring it back with the hole stopped up and try to pass it off, with a clear intent to deceive. That is fraud. My dear Goat, I'm afraid the grand jury will get after you if you are not more careful about little things of this sort."

Moral: The fable teaches that the moral quality of a business transaction often depends on the view you take of it.

---

[1] Adapted from "The Rabbit and the Goat," in *Life*, October 8, 1885, p. 208.

8

Dear Ethical
Practice Board:

The Golden Rule is that there are no golden rules.   (G. B. Shaw)

In its existence an ethical practice committee receives many requests for advice on matters of ethics from conscientious association members. Most members are seeking direction on a particular practice pattern to avoid possible confrontation with an ethics infraction at a later date. Some are gathering information in preparation for reporting on another member and want to be certain they are on solid ground before taking action. A few try to trip-up an ethics board in one of its previous findings in hopes of helping a friend who was sanctioned at some earlier time. By and large, however, the requests express the genuine concern of professionals who want to do what is right and are willing to seek and follow the advice of the group monitoring the ethical behavior of their association.

As requests describe very real concerns of professional practitioners, the committee is obligated to afford each request the full attention and reasoned deliberation of the ethics monitors. But that is the easy part. The difficult part is to be certain of the question being asked, the circumstances surrounding the specific issue being addressed, and that the answer is not ambiguous. Equally important is to recognize that the writer may be requesting a written answer as an insurance policy against a possible ethics citation at some date in the future.

The advisories, as they are most often called, that are generated by ethics committees have a way of becoming the "standard of practice" in a particular situation. Recall that the AMA has only seven Principles to its Code of Ethics, and the Opinions offered by members of the Committee on Ethical and Judicial Affairs make up the accepted standard of practice conduct. Preparation and opinions must be written with great care. In the case of the AMA these published reports become the interpretation of standards against which practitioners measure their own ethical behavior. In the case of most other professions the advisory opinions are between the ethics committee and the correspondent, unless the committee elects to publish the advice as a general interpretation. Interpretive reports allow for a code of ethics to be less detailed. The principles are stated in more global terms and are fleshed out later through statements of interpretation, or advisories.

Some professions develop codes of ethical conduct that are very general in nature, lacking the specificity of other codes in the belief that not every situation can be addressed in a code document. In this case, the code document is used primarily to publicize the profession's values to the public. As ethical issues arise or as requests are received for a specific interpretation, the code is explained. Advisories and the results of deliberations surrounding particular ethical transgressions become a part of ethics code interpretation. This practice helps to assure consistency within the ethics committee's findings.

A few professional organizations regularly publish advisories in their professional bulletin to keep the topic of ethics current and consistent with its members and as a method of educating the membership concerning possible ethics indiscretions. The material in this chapter was adapted from letters received by professional ethics committees. The letters are abridged and a certain degree of journalistic license has been taken to ensure that none can be traced to a specific individual or incident. The intent of including the material is to present real examples of issues concerning members of professional associations, and some of the difficulties faced by an ethics committee in providing guidance to the correspondent.

ADVISORIES

Request for Action

Dear Committee on Ethics:

I am an audiologist employed by a large hospital that dispenses hearing aids. Recently the CEO got a letter from the [state hearing aid dealers' licensing board] Consumer Protection Division requesting that we issue a check for $645.00 to [a client we had put a hearing aid on] because [he/she] doesn't want the hearing aid we sold. [The client] says that we used tactics to get [him/her] to buy the instrument and that [he/she] told us [he/she] had never wanted it in the first place, but that we put it on [him/her] and took the money. I don't know for sure what . . . [was] . . . told to the Consumer Protection office, but that's sort of what they said in the letter to my boss.

Of course this isn't true, but now my boss wants a full explanation of what we do down here about selling hearing aids and [the boss] wants to pay [the client] back the money. I think this is wrong because we didn't do what was claimed, and besides the client has had the hearing aid for 10 months.

I'm afraid that if I don't do what my boss asks I might be terminated. I don't think it is ethical for [the CEO] to ask this. Also I think to give the client a refund is unethical and a blight against me and audiology. Can you help me by writing to my boss and telling him/her this is unethical.

Thank you for your assistance.

Before reading further, attempt to draft an advisory yourself. Select the issues you feel are important to the letter writer and within your area of expertise. Draft an answer and then compare it to the actual ethics committee's position.

The Committee's Approach

Here's how one ethics committee managed the letter. First, the ethics committee recognized that it could correspond with the letter-writer and ask for specifics surrounding the evaluation and fitting of the hearing aid, a description or copy of the department's dispensing policies and procedures, and special stipulations of the hearing aid dealers' licensing statute that might be applicable. The committee might then determine whether a deviation from the written policy occurred and submit a response to the audiologist based on its interpretation of those requisites.

That approach is a time-consuming process that often unintentionally intimidates the letter-writer. It also rests heavily on materials sent to the committee by the correspondent. These materials may or may not be complete.

As a second option, the committee could simply base an answer on the letter as submitted. If the committee elected the second approach (which is preferable), some caution in developing the answer would be required. The letter-writer's contention that the CEO is unethical is not the business of the committee and any reference to that issue should be judiciously avoided. However, there is really nothing unethical about refunding a client's money if the situation warrants it, regardless of the stipulations of the law that might, for instance, indicate that responsibility to refund ceases after 30 days. Neither is there anything unethical in the act of *not* refunding it under the circumstances as described. The writer could be told all of that.

The refund may not be a good business decision, however, as in this case the client had the hearing aid for 10 months. Conversely, the CEO may think that having a satisfied customer, an ally in the field, is indeed good for the hospital and $645.00, or some lesser amount, is not an expensive way to get it. Refunding might, nonetheless, be an admission of a guilt that is not there, thus undermining the audiologist and the department. In any case, corporate decisions are also not the responsibility of the ethics committee. Finally, the CEO's request for a description of the department's policies and procedures concerning hearing aid dispensing is reasonable and certainly justified, but again beyond the committee's responsibility for comment.

An answer to the writer based on the information contained in the letter, therefore, would probably merely point out that from the facts presented, there is no evidence to substantiate that the audiologist is in violation of the code of ethics with reference to the specific incident described, and further indicate that it is not within the purview of the association's ethics committee to monitor the ethics practices of those not under its jurisdiction. The letter should be concise and unambiguous.

Request for Advice on Restraint of Trade

Dear Ethics Committee:

I am a partner in a speech/language pathology practice with one other [person] until the [end of the month]. We have been together for 11 years. I joined the practice 11 years ago. My partner had me sign a contract at the time which I signed readily because I was young and eager to begin seeing clients.

Now I want to leave the partnership and start my own office. Some of my clients want to stay with me, but my partner says I can't have their records and that if I take the clients away [he/she] will sue me. [He/She] says I signed a contract 11 years ago restricting me from opening up a practice within 25 miles. I didn't know I did that, but I was shown where it said it in the contract. My lawyer is checking to see if that is still legal.

What I want to know from the ethics board is if it is unethical for my former partner to limit the services of those people who want to come with me. Also, isn't it unethical for [my former partner] to keep the records? Don't those records belong to the client? Do you think it's ethical for [him/her] to keep me from making a living in my field?

Please write [him/her] a letter saying it is unethical and a restraint of trade to keep me from opening an office and making a living.

Again, it would be helpful to think through your own approach to this request and to draft an answer before looking at what the committee would do. There are a couple of sensitive areas in this one, so be thoughtful.

The Committee's Advice

First, the committee cannot respond to the partner saying anything is **unethical** based on the information contained in the correspondent's letter. The committee can, however, write to the correspondent indicating that if the correspondent wishes to take a formal action against the partner citing a violation of the code of ethics, the committee would be happy to deliberate it.

On the assumption that the partner did, in fact, refuse to relinquish client's records to the clients who requested them there may be grounds for noncompliance with the code. That cannot be realistically judged until information is received from both parties.

The committee could comment further on the matter of the records. The records *do* belong to the clients, and they should be allowed to obtain copies (perhaps for a fee) and do what they wish with them. It should also be pointed out to the correspondent that the partner did not refuse to give the records to the *clients*, according to the information in the letter. The correspondent was told of possible suit **if he/she** took the clients away from the office.

The committee should not comment on the matter of restraint of trade. The issue of a "restrictive clause" is better handled by an attorney.

As in the first example, the response should be brief and to the point. The writer has asked specific questions of the committee and these should be addressed without fueling a fire. So far, at least, it does not appear that an ethics transgression has been committed.

Request for Approval of Advertising Copy

Dear Ethics Committee:

Enclosed you will find a copy of an advertisement I plan to run in the [local shopping mall] advertiser. Several of my colleagues and my wife have thought it to be unethical. I would appreciate the committee's approval before I submit it. Please answer quickly because I am in a "dog fight" with my competition, and the holidays are getting closer.

The following copy, which has been edited only to protect confidentiality, was attached to the letter:

SILENT NIGHT, SILENT NIGHT?
THIS HOLIDAY SEASON WILL YOUR NIGHTS
ALL BE SILENT BECAUSE YOU CAN'T HEAR THE
STRAINS OF THE SEASON'S CHRISTMAS SONGS?

MAYBE IT'S TIME YOU GAVE [hearing aid brand]
A TRY

HEAR ALL THE BEAUTIFUL SOUNDS OF THIS
JOYFUL SEASON.

HAVE A CUSTOM SELECTED HEARING AID
IN TIME FOR CHRISTMAS—
CALL 555-5555
OR JUST STOP BY FOR A TRIAL
123 SOME STREET
ANYWHERE SHOPPING MALL
EVERYONE WILL HAVE A MERRY CHRISTMAS
All major credit cards accepted

Try developing a response. Remember what the writer is asking of the ethics committee. Don't overdo your response.

The Committee's Response

Basing an answer on the Codes of Ethics of ASHA and the AAA, the committee would have to judge that the enclosed ad copy does not violate the code of either organization. Whether the copy is in good taste is another issue and one that is difficult to discuss. With regard to preferences, professional associations believe that ad copy should enhance professional image and not belong to the broad genre of hucksterism. Ads should reflect the caliber of other copy found in the locale, as well as conform to the spirit of the practitioner's code of ethics.

Unless a professional organization has developed guidelines that clearly indicate prohibitions on certain phrasing, fonts, ad size, and so on, a great deal of latitude will have to be allowed concerning the matter of preference. As long as an advertisement does not mislead, misrepresent, or deceive, it will probably be judged ethical. Discussion related to preference should be avoided in creating advisories.

Request for a Graduate School Recommendation

Dear Sir/Madame:

I am a graduating college senior and am interested in going into speech therapy or audiology. I have applied to the Graduate School at [John Doeville University] but have recently been told that it is not an accredited graduate program and that several of the professors have been in trouble with ethics in the past. Now I don't know what to do. In a way I still want to go there anyway.

I would appreciate your sending information about the school and about the professors. Their names are: [3 names given]. Also please advise me what is best for me to do about school.

Thank you.

The facts are: (1) the program is not accredited (by the Educational and Training Board of ASHA), (2) each of the professors named in the correspondence has been reported for an alleged ethics infraction within the past 3 years. One was reprimanded with no publication of charge or finding. Two were sanctioned more severely, (3) the infraction and the sanction were published. Develop an answer to the writer before you read how the committee responded.

The Committee's Answer

Dear Whoever:

The Ethical Practice Board is charged with interpreting the Code of Ethics of the Association and monitoring the professional conduct of its members to assure compliance with the Principles and Rules stated in the Code. Although most of the workings of the Board are confidential, some violations carry a sanction that requires notification by means of publication in a widely read professional journal. Notification of an ethics violation was published in the [month] issue of [Journal] regarding two of the individuals mentioned in your letter. Quoting in part:

> John Doe was judged by the Ethical Practice Board to be in noncompliance with Principle [X], Rule [Y] of the Code of Ethics for failure to....

> Sanction is suspension of membership for a three-month period ending July 15, 1992....

> Mary Rey was judged by the Ethical Practice Board to be in

noncompliance with Principle [K], Rule [A] of the Code of Ethics for participating in a situation judged by the Board to be not in the best interest of the person(s) being served at the time.

Sanction is suspension of the Certificate of Clinical Competence in Speech-Language Pathology for a six-month period ending October 1, 1992, after which time the Certificate will be restored without additional demonstration of qualification.

Information concerning the accreditation status of the academic program should be requested of the Chairman of the Department. You may also wish to research the ranking of the program and the institution through your local library.

CAVEAT EMPTOR REVISITED

The following letter, although fictitious, represents an occurrence with serious ethics overtones. The situation described in the letter is based on facts.

The Situation

Dear Ethics Board:

Recently I was a participant on a cruise sponsored by [one of the hearing aid manufacturers]. Even though I was selected for the cruise because I purchased almost the required number of hearing aids and contributed the difference in money from my personal account, I believe some unethical things were done that you should know about. I don't always agree with some of our ethics code, but sometimes I think people go too far.

The boat was very nice and [hearing aid company] was an excellent host. There was lots of food and drinks. My spouse and I don't drink so that didn't bother us one way or another. But we eat a lot, and we ate a lot on the cruise, but that didn't bother us either because we figured it was paid for out of our pocket and from the [hearing] aids we bought.

It was a good time. We swam and sat in the sun and danced. It must have cost [the company] a big sum of money. There were a lot of people on board. The [Company] planned several educational sessions which dealt with their product. Most of the sessions were presented by audiologists well known in the hearing aid field for their research, one or two talks were about marketing and sales and were given by dispensing audiologists, and one talk was by a [Company] official. The talks were well attended.

One morning in one of the meeting rooms there were Styrofoam® boxes on the table in front of each chair; maybe 60 boxes, maybe more. On the top of the box was a label with my name and address on it.

Other boxes had other names and addresses.

Inside the box were two [hearing aid company] BTE hearing aids and an invoice in the amount of $600 made out to my office. There was also an explanation that if I came to the front of the room I could pick up $200 in cash and the invoice would be redrawn for $400 instead of the $600. Even though I declined to participate, when I got back to my office there was an invoice in my mail for the two BTEs stating that $400 was due.

It seems to me that [Company] is doing something unethical here, and that the audiologists who participate in the offer are also in a conflict of interest situation. I could name names here, but I choose not to do that at this time. I would like advice, however, about the nature of this episode as far as the ethics of [Company] is concerned.

Thank-you for your consideration.

The Ethics Position

The ethics of the company is not under the jurisdiction of a professional association.

The situation described by the audiologist is not a new one. Cruises, foreign travel, junkets in guise as educational seminars, and the like are part of the history of the relationship between hearing aid manufacturers and audiologists. History alone does not place such activities any less in opposition to the ethics of a profession, however.

These offerings are merely a marketing tactic of a higher order than the hospitality suites and parties sponsored at annual professional convention meetings. In most aspects they are similar to what pharmaceutical manufacturing companies provide for medical practitioners. The reasons for the practice are identical in both instances. In the case of the relationship between the Pharmaceuticals and the AMA, however, the United States Senate became keenly interested and has extracted an agreement from each limiting the kinds of "gifts" that can be offered and accepted.

It is not likely that the federal government will look into the relationships audiologists maintain with hearing aid manufacturers, because the federal government does not provide financial support for hearing aids under the Medicare program. The rationale for government involvement in Pharmaceutical–AMA relations was simply that because the government, through its Medicare reimbursement for medicines and drugs, was reeling in response to the rapid and tremendous rise in the cost of medications charged to the program legislators had a right and a responsibility to curtail those costs. They wanted the practices dropped. They got their way.

The investigation's consequence to the AMA was the embarrassment of having the expensive trips and other perks made public. The AMA initiated drafting guidelines to divert opinion from the appearance of conflicts of interest, and the pharmaceuticals quickly joined in support of the new, less pressured, and less expensive relationship.

What role state-sponsored health programs will take in lowering costs is a matter that still looms on the horizon. Indications are that some states are beginning to question the cost to state coffers when a provider clearly takes advantage of value incentive offers, but fails to pass the savings along. If interest is tweaked and the states begin to look with disfavor on the current cost of hearing aids, it is a safe bet that lavish giving by hearing aid manufacturers will come under fire, and the professional conduct of audiologists will also be scrutinized.

Still another concern with the foregoing letter and the situation described may even involve the Internal Revenue Service. Large companies such as pharmaceuticals and hearing aid manufacturers are required to report the value of gifts which exceed a certain amount and to indicate the recipient. It is likely that the audiologist(s) participating in the cruise as described above will receive an MI-1099 (Miscellaneous Income form) from the sponsor of the cruise. The amount specified will be the dollar value of the trip and must be claimed as personal income by the recipient. The giver of the trip claims it as an expense. The question arises once again, "In whose best interest was the whole thing, anyway?"

As if the implications and applications of all those concerns aren't enough, there is still the matter of ethics to be considered. The letter specifically addresses the ethics of the company sponsoring the cruise, as well as the involvement of the audiologists who participated in the marketing scheme, bought the hearing aids, and accepted the $200 cash payment. As a passenger on the cruise who did not accept the hearing aid offer, the writer of the letter has excluded him/herself as a practitioner possibly in noncompliance with a professional code of ethics. It has obviously not occurred to the individual that the mere act of being a passenger under the circumstances *may* be a violation of ethics principles.

The company appears to have obeyed the Golden Rule. The technique used is often referred to as "captive marketing." In this instance it was a well-thought-out scheme to offer a cruise in exchange for the purchase of a specified quantity of instruments; an on-board product sales pitch; $200 in cash in exchange for the purchase of two hearing aids for which $400 would be owed; and the not-so-remote possibility that the cruisers would reciprocate for the good time with continued purchases.

The audiologists who participated may or may not feel good

about the offer from the business viewpoint. From the ethics position it is anything but good. At the very least there is an *appearance* of a conflict of interest. At the very worst there actually is a conflict of interest and it may be demonstrated to exist among the audiologists who participated in the cruise and who accepted the offer tied to the hearing aids.

Somewhere in the continuum the ethics monitors would consider the act of taking the $200, and finally there is the knowledge that when the letter is answered at least one audiologist will know there is a possible ethics violation. Further, that audiologist has knowledge of who on board may be in violation and has elected not to make their names known. That in itself is a violation of the professional code. The matter is not simple.

Caveat emptor is a caution not given lightly. It applies to all buyers. It has special meaning in today's market and special application to today's professional health care practitioners. As more public attention is given to the quality of services provided by professionals, the number of advisories sent to ethics committees of professional organizations will increase in response. Ethics monitors will be called on not only to monitor ongoing behavior, but to advise practitioners concerning potential areas of noncompliance with the dictates of a code of ethical conduct. This may very well be the measure of the sensitivity a professional exhibits for the difference between business and professional ethics.

9

Why All the
Fuss Over Ethics?

*Where observation is concerned, chance favors only the prepared
mind.*   (Louis Pasteur)

Most behavior transgressions violate some aspect of what most
people believe to be the principles of goodness, virtue, and
ethics. The very persons that everyone grew up trusting, for example
the minister, the doctor, the sports hero, the policeman, the college
professor, et cetera, are falling, according to the news media, far short
of traditional moral expectations.

Practitioners in most professional fields seemingly are becoming
defensive and are fearful of not being trusted. They are beginning to
look toward outwardly improving their conduct. Professions, even
small ones such as audiology and speech-language pathology, are
developing and revising codes of professional ethics. Ethics codes are
once again being publicized.

Traditionally, audiology and speech-language pathology have
not devoted much publicity to the code of ethics associated with their
major national organization until recently. Although the written code
of ethics governing the behavior of these professions has existed for
decades, the number of alleged violations of the codes has been relatively small in comparison to the size of the associations. The number
of proven noncompliances with the codes is even smaller. This does
not necessarily describe an organization whose membership is non-

chalant about ethical practices, nor does it indicate a lack of commitment to ethics enforcement. Likewise, a low incidence of noncompliance with a code of ethics should not be construed to indicate a collection of practitioners who do everything with goodness and virtue.

Ethics is simply not something that has commanded open attention and activity in the past. Few people are required to take coursework in ethics during their academic preparation. Additionally, not many individuals are willing to *report* an apparent violator of the ethics code. As a result, professional ethics is relegated to an individual level governed solely by the goodness of one's character, one's virtuousness, and one's sense of what is right. Substantial, but not always enough.

Speech-language pathology and audiology practitioners as a group need ethics education if for no other reason than that they are professionals who are not required to chalk up formal coursework in the area. Some do, but many do not, appreciate the need for or the implications of a set of association rules governing the behavior of members.

ASHA's code has been revised and finely tuned by the association's ethics monitors to reflect the nuances of modern practice. The attitude of nonprofessionals who conduct business with the practitioners of speech-language pathology and audiology has changed as well. Similarly, the potential conflict of interest atmosphere surrounding professional conventions and, therefore open to public perception, is more controlled than in previous times.

Nonetheless, there are the ever-present temptations to dilute the principles of professionalism to whatever degree possible. As with the AMA, all professions must be wary if professionalism in the traditional sense is to survive. Change is inevitable, but when the tail begins to wag the dog, restructuring becomes a must.

THE PERKS FROM THEN TO NOW

In the 1950s, 60s, and most of the 70s the annual ASHA conventions offered manufacturer-sponsored open houses. These functions were usually attended by both audiologists and speech-language pathologists who gave no thought to the appearance of conflict of interest in that atmosphere of "free-loading" from the maker of a product with which the professional was directly involved. It was simply the thing to do. Everybody did it. Nobody cared. Many of the manufacturers' "hospitality suites" were talked about for weeks following the convention. The ethics of it all was never discussed and was not an issue.

In those days it is unlikely that the hospitality activity had any influence on what audiologists or speech pathologists did with products when they went home, but one can never be sure. Most who spirited the hospitality suites had little influence on institutional selection and purchase of hearing aids anyway. Few audiologists were in private practice and therefore not in a posture to be selective about instrument buying. Influence peddling by the suppliers of products was broad and largely not effective.

Regardless of this, before long, limits were placed on the flexibility previously enjoyed by manufacturers of products. The number of hospitality suites at convention meetings was drastically curtailed by edict of those individuals in the (then) American Speech and Hearing Association having the vision to see the possible appearance of a conflict of interest and the potential effect of influence peddling on the image of the profession.

When the abundance of hospitality suites for convention attendees dwindled as a result of limitations the enticements changed. Hospitality suites were replaced by lavish dinners in the convention city, but not in the convention hotel—offered only for select groups. The approach became more targeted. Gifts for program chiefs and staff began to arrive at holiday time.

Ultimately, inducements to remain highly interested in a particular product were elevated to providing expense-paid foreign trips for audiologists. In the early days, these trips were by invitation only and offered one or two times each year. Lots of folks went. Sometimes audiologists were even included in groups of hearing aid specialists. But, in the early days of trips, audiologists were enticed by an aura of continuing education and exchange of scientific information that hung loosely over each sojourn. This approach in the guise of respectability went a degree beyond targeted. The targets became captive.

Another thing has changed since the 70s, also. Today audiologists are more influential in institutional product acquisition matters, and more audiologists are in private practice or associated with a private dispensing activity. Industry marketing can now take better aim, with greater opportunity for hitting the bulls-eye.

Trips continue today as an enticement to use more of a particular product. Now, however, foreign trips must be "won" and are linked to a volume purchase of the product or some other value-incentive program. The end result is the same. It continues to be a marketing practice by product manufacturers. They are good at it and they should be. It is still, as in the 50s and 60s, influence peddling and it comes in many forms. All such practices are tailored by major industry to move products into the marketplace, and all infringe to varying degrees on professional ethics.

Because of their dependency on hearing aids as vital in the provision of hearing health care audiologists must recognize that they represent a handsome target for influence peddling. Some do realize it. Some don't. Many who do, downplay the need for ethics by knowing that *they* are good people and believing that *they* simply could *never* be influenced. A few don't quite understand the implications that influence peddling, the appearance of conflicts of interest, the acceptance of value incentives, etc. have on the public image of a profession.

To a great extent the lack of sophistication in understanding and appreciating professional ethics is not the fault of the practitioner. The relationship between hearing aid product manufacturers and audiologists, for instance, has since the 1950s been one that has seen toleration, and perhaps even *expectation* that, some level of "gift giving" such as that which began with hospitality suites at annual meetings and today is disguised in quantity discount programs and travel incentive packages. No one in the profession has ever objected. The arrangement, the practice, and the expectations are quite similar to the physician–pharmaceutical manufacturers' relationship described in an earlier chapter. The fate of that arrangement is sealed, and at this juncture, it can best be used as a teaching example and as a guide for other professions in dealings with the perks of commercial enterprises.

The manufacturers who offer these enticements are not solely to blame, either. Business is business, and their business is to sell products. Put another way, their business is to influence people, any people, to buy their product instead of the goods of a competitor. If a case of cognac given to the right person will help make that sale, a case will be given. If a $7,000 trip to Liverpool will help ensure higher sales volume from hearing and speech centers, a trip will be offered. The temptation possibilities are virtually endless.

OTHER ETHICS CONCERNS

Events are happening in other sectors of the speech-language pathology professions with regard to ethics, as well. There is growing concern, for example, that individuals intent on being called *doctor* are enrolling in nonaccredited doctoral degree programs, mail-order degree mills, or obtaining a doctoral degree in a major area unrelated to the management of communicative disorders. The ethics worry, obviously, is that individuals who sport degrees of this type are willfully misleading the public, are being deceptive, and may be found guilty of violating the public trust.

The problem of fee-splitting is yet another ethics concern. Audiologists as well as speech-language pathologists have for many years provided services in a physician's office. Some do this on a full-time basis, others as a part-time activity. Compensation for the speech-language or audiology person in a part-time arrangement is often based in a percentage of the amount collected by the physician. The simple term for this may be fee-splitting. Justification for the physician to keep a portion is generally based in the expense of space and supplies. But the key word is "collected."

The ethics of this type of arrangement are questionable because it is not defensible to pay only for services for which funds are collected. Some audiology practitioners insist that payment percentage be based on the amount *billed*, rather than the amount collected. The reasons for this are obvious. The ethics, however, are only slightly easier to defend.

The issues become more complicated and even less clear ethically in the case of audiologists who dispense hearing aids in physicians' offices and somehow split the collection for the instrument sale. There is also the questionable ethics of the situation in which an audiologist is told by an employing physician to "just test bone conduction in the left ear, please," or "don't explain the test results to my patients. I'll do that." The audiologist who allows this to continue may be criticized for not assuming the professional responsibility required of an audiologist, and may even be cited for noncompliance with a code rule.

Again however, although ignorance of the rules is not a valid defense, the doer is not solely to blame. The physician has never been challenged in this aspect of practice and the audiologist or speech-language pathologist has never been exposed to directed ethics teaching. It is, then, more the fault of the fields of speech and hearing for not having placed ethics at the forefront in the past. But that is changing because of the heightened sensitivity to ethics. Every professional needs to be taught more about ethics. The time for that is now. Such study won't answer all the shortcomings involved in product dispensing by a professional, but it is a step toward a better understanding of what can go wrong.

It would be presumptuous to assume that the full duty of a professional to a patient, client, co-worker, profession, and society will always be covered in clear fashion by ethical, legal, and moral teachings designating acceptable behavior. Reality is not always what is expected. Worse yet, the reality of a situation may often mandate compliance with a host of rules that might contradict ethical conduct, among other things.

Add to that recognition, the demands of a rapidly changing society wherein good for goodness sake, right for the sake of righteousness, and morality for the preservation of mankind appear destined to move from Cadillac-to-Chevrolet class. All the answers aren't in yet and perhaps all the questions haven't yet been asked, but some examples of the state-of-the-art in this regard are evident throughout society and the professions, because everyone is making a fuss over ethics.

THE ENGINEERING PROFESSION

For the engineering profession, attention given to anxieties over ethics is clearly illustrated by the dilemmas faced in the NASA space shuttle disasters, the Hyatt-Regency skywalk catastrophe, and the McManus River Bridge collapse in Connecticut, all of which received national publicity.

At the same time, but less publicized, a physician's decision to proceed with an experimental treatment or nurses' decisions to strike against an employer or countermand doctors' orders represent professional challenges equal in magnitude to the moral stresses that faced the engineers involved with the aforementioned failures. These dilemmas involve loyalty to patients, obligations to protect the health, welfare, and safety of society, a duty to preserve the values of a profession, and an obligation to respect the decisions of policymakers and those in authority. In short, they involve the ethics of professions.

Within the professions, an awareness of the need for enhanced ethics sensitivity has created a momentum for professional organizations to move in the direction of a focused emphasis on the values espoused by each. Perhaps, for example, as a direct result of the engineering disasters, engineering schools are providing students the opportunity to achieve a more well-rounded educational experience offering them an orientation to the current status, practice, and problems of the engineering profession and how it interfaces with society. In other words, engineering students are now being directly exposed to the ethics of their profession.

The engineering profession, as a matter of fact, provides an excellent ancillary example in a discussion of all the fuss about ethics. At the outset, one needs to understand that the term "engineer" is one of the most misapplied nouns in the English language. For instance, there is the so-called sanitation engineer, the building engineer, the systems engineer, the telecommunications engineer, the audio engineer, the grounds engineer, the genetics engineer, the locomotive engineer, and even the management engineer, to name several. None of these is really an engineer in the true definition of the word.

The word *engineer* is derived from the word "ingenuity" and relates to the concept of design. Precisely speaking, engineering is the application of science and mathematics to the properties of matter and the sources of energy in nature to render them useful to human beings, machines, structures, products, and systems.

Engineers are involved in virtually every constructed object in our lives; they design the structural members for our dams, skyscrapers, and bridges; the systems bringing water into our homes and taking waste away; they design microchips, artificial organs for the human

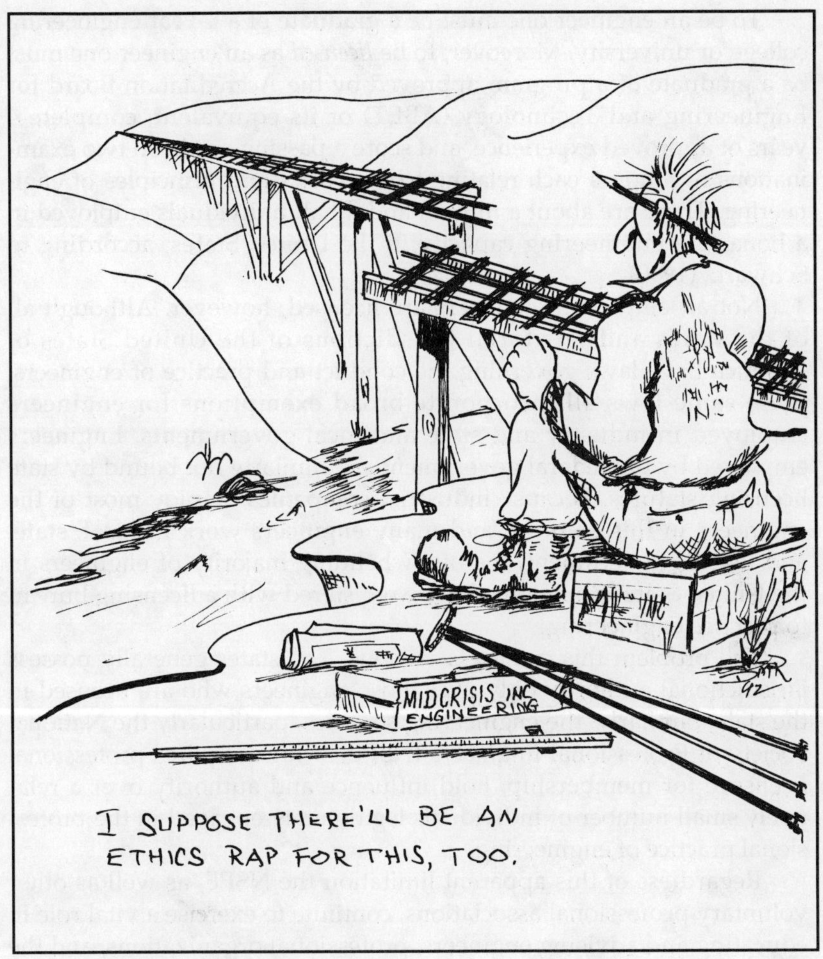

body, prostheses, surgical instruments, electronic circuitry, highways, and so on. They are applied scientists—design professionals. Unfortunately, technologists, technicians, equipment operators, broadcasters, laborers, efficiency experts, and many others are granted the title of "engineer" by their employer regardless of whether they have the education, experience, competence, or license to be an engineer by strict definition.

One reason for this misappropriation of title is that to be an engineer is to wear a cloak of respectability, and everybody wants respect and to be a professional. Recall from Chapter 1 that trade associations make an effort to develop a code of ethics as a public statement of their principles, albeit that their attempt is not frequently successful.

To be an engineer one must be a graduate of a 4-year engineering college or university. Moreover, to be *licensed* as an engineer one must be a graduate of a program approved by the Accreditation Board for Engineering and Technology (ABET) or its equivalent, complete 4 years of approved experience, and score a passing grade on two examinations of 8 hours each relating to the basics and principles of engineering. There are about a million-and-a-half individuals employed in a bona fide engineering capacity in the United States, according to Schwartz (1990).

Not all employed engineers are licensed, however. Although all of the states and territorial jurisdictions of the United States of America have laws governing the conduct and practice of engineers, these same laws all incorporate broad exemptions for engineers employed in industry and state and local governments. Engineers employed by the federal government are similarly not bound by state licensing statutes. Because industrial companies employ most of the engineers in this country, and many engineers work in local, state, and federal government, the overwhelming majority of engineers in the United States do not need to be registered with a licensing bureau to practice engineering.

The problem this creates is obvious. The states generally possess jurisdictional authority only over those engineers who are licensed in the state. Similarly, the engineering societies, particularly the National Society of Professional Engineers (NSPE), which requires professional licensure for membership, hold influence and authority over a relatively small number of individuals legitimately engaged in the professional practice of engineering.

Regardless of this apparent limitation the NSPE, as well as other voluntary professional associations, continue to exercise a vital role in educating and advising engineers, professional organizations, and the public on matters involving the professional ethics of engineering. These groups are also known to play a major role in disciplining members, insofar as possible, in matters of unethical or unprofessional conduct. The NSPE has since its establishment in 1934 promoted the Code of Ethics for Professional Engineers (Schwartz, 1990). Their code contains a Preamble, Fundamental Canons, and Rules of Practice. It is a frequently cited code within and outside the profession of engineering.

Ethics is important to the association and to engineers in general. However, in the matter of discipline, as a private voluntary organization the NSPE is somewhat constrained in its ability to sanction practicing engineers. First, its authority only extends to those who are members. As membership in the society requires a license, and because the great majority of practicing engineers are exempt from licensing by virtue of their employment, the society does not have hard disciplinary authority over a very large number of people. Second, the most extreme penalty that a voluntary professional society such as the NSPE can impose is expulsion from the society. The effect of this sanction has limited impact, because membership in the society is not a legal requirement for practice.

Despite these seemingly severe limitations, the NSPE is active in taking disciplinary action against its members who have engaged in unethical or unprofessional conduct and in publishing the results of their actions in society periodicals. Publication of actions against unethical conduct is the most useful and effective function that voluntary professional associations can provide in disciplining members. Publicizing the actions among peers sends an important message to the membership that the organization believes the ethical conduct of its professional members is more important than just words on parchment.

SIMILARITIES TO SPEECH-LANGUAGE PATHOLOGY/AUDIOLOGY

Engineering, like speech-language pathology and audiology, has become increasingly specialized and sub-subspecialized. At one time, a professional engineer practiced in a broad spectrum of areas: civil, mechanical, and electrical. Today that is different. Most modern engineers have narrowed their focus to a specific substrate within one of the three broad categories. In this regard the profession is similar to speech-language pathology and audiology, in which practitioners usually become expert in a specialty area within the discipline.

The ethics concern raised here is one that questions the validity of the message sent to the consumer by a practitioner who holds the Certificate of Clinical Competence. The certificate, after all, indicates that the holder is competent in all clinical aspects of the practice represented by the credential. Whether such a broad announcement is misleading and therefore in conflict with ethics stipulations is at least worth considering. Perhaps it is even sufficient motivation to reinstate discussions of the need for specialty certification within speech-language pathology and audiology.

A case in point might be that of an individual employed as a clinical fellow in speech-language pathology who, immediately following completion of the fellowship year, accepts a position as Director of Communication Disorder Services in a satellite hospital program on the outskirts of the city. The person's CFY experience focused mainly on management of adult neurogenic disorders. The satellite program is devoted predominantly to laryngectomized patients. If there is an ethics question here, it revolves around the high probability that the neophyte practitioner has not amassed sufficient real-world experience to function well in such a responsible position, in addition to which award of the clinical credential may be an overstatement of the fact. Is accepting such a position deceitful and not representative of the person's management or clinical skills and therefore unethical? Perhaps.

On the one hand, it is unlikely that a clinical fellowship year provides experience in the management, budgetary, hiring, and termination skills necessary to the position of program director. The credential achieved only attests to *clinical competence* and has little to say about areas beyond the bounds of clinical experience. Within the area of clinical experience the question becomes one of focus. Is the practitioner guilty of deception by undertaking to manage a program devoted to laryngectomees when experience was gained predominantly in neurogenic disorders?

On the other hand, why should an individual be penalized for accepting an opportunity for personal growth and development? Can a code of ethics that requires individuals avoid practicing in areas for which they do not possess experience and training also support the credibility of a clinical certificate which attests to competence in *all* clinical areas? The ASHA Code (1992) only indicates that individuals shall provide services in the area for which they are credentialed. The Certificate of Clinical Competence, then, says to the public that the holder is capable of working with all types of speech-language disorders. Is this misleading? And who is at fault? The practitioner? the code? the association? the requirements for possession of the certificate?

It is reasonable to argue that seekers of the certificate are required to accumulate experience with a variety of disorders so that the above example would not be likely to occur. What then of the certified practitioner with 5 years of experience exclusively in the management of swallowing disorders in a medical institution who opens a private practice and takes on three laryngectomees as the first patients? Are the consumers likely to think they are getting something they actually are not getting? Very likely.

As another example, audiologists may function in the office of a physician, who may not allow the audiologist sufficient time to complete a traditional hearing test. This is especially so for repeat tests, and it is not unusual for the hypothetical physician to request a partial test such as bone conduction at 500 and 1000 Hz only or to request a test only of the left ear. There may be times when a request of this nature is justified, but there are also occasions when such a request restricts the quality of audiologic services provided. Is there a risk of ethics violation in instances like this? Perhaps.

PRESERVATION OF THE PROFESSIONS
BY PROFESSIONALS

There is no question that corruption is in the headlines daily. It seems, too, that under every stone there is not just one worm, but an infestation. But perhaps worst of all is that society is willing to tolerate the situation—if, in fact, it *is* willing. There is also no argument that ethics as a topic of discussion is getting more attention today than in past decades, and further, that with increased attention to what is right, the tolerance threshold of most society members shrinks.

The reasons for this are varied. In some instances society's members are personally involved and are profiting from dishonesty and corruption. Some members of society are weak and apathetic and afraid to take courageous steps to stop the raging rip-offs. Some have no values other than money. A large number seem content in the belief that as long as reasonable ethical standards are observed personally, there is no need to feel responsible for the conduct of others. Finally, there are those who do not believe corruption is all that bad. The longer society lives with deviant conduct, the more it begins to appear all right.

Yet, deep in the viscera of most people there is a sense that these comparatively mild symptoms of ethical transgressions are but the first hue of a deeper fever. If permitted to worsen unchecked, corruption and other unethical conduct will render a United States of America teeming with violent crimes, senseless demonstrations against the system, and a lust for wealth and power. The effect will be to leave cherished principles and finer instincts of society as the first casualties. Without a strong foundation of ethics, laws cannot become and will not remain effective. Without honesty, freedom is not safe. Without freedom, it is unsafe to be honest. Ask Solzhenitsyn! Ponder the plight of Sakharov!

As professions move into the 21st century professional societies are obligated to ensure that their members become acutely aware of the ethical, moral, and legal components of not only the decision-making process, but the process of preserving the public trust as well. There are common ethical issues emerging all the time. No matter what profession is involved, engineering, medicine, law, speech-language pathology, audiology, there is a common bond. Self-regulation of professions demands intellectual expertise, along with the provision of services to ensure the optimal functioning of society. It is crucial that their professional members provide for and abide by the ethical conduct of their associations.

The issues involved in professional ethics are complex and dynamic—particularly in professions that are comparatively young and still experiencing growing pains. There is cause for great hope among those professions that embrace a code of ethics with sincerity. The success of professions depends on the ability of seasoned practitioners to see the need for control of ethical conduct among professionals and on their willingness to accept individual responsibility to preserve it. Awareness of ethical conduct as it relates to the professions must be heightened, perhaps through sensitivity training, perhaps through the formal teaching of ethics in all, not just a few, professional graduate education programs.

THE TEACHING OF ETHICS

Philosophy departments in some universities have initiated applied units of study in which discipline-specific approaches to analyzing ethics strategies are presented. Others continue to offer only the philosophical perspectives that involve analyses that provide students with little more than aspirational goals. Unfortunately, professional ethics is not as abstract as these philosophical exercises would suggest. Professional ethics is multifaceted. Some schools provide courses for students enrolled in professional programs, but they are largely elective offerings, and the formal teaching of professional ethics remains underemphasized.

Despite the apparent need for schools and professional societies to assume an interdisciplinary role in developing common strategies for providing preprofessionals with knowledge in ethics, there are still those who believe that ethics cannot be taught. Some argue that medical ethics, for example, can only be taught by living it and expressing it in daily actions (Wright, 1987). Some, in the field of engineering, believe that the profession is "value free." Their argument, however unconvincingly, is that engineers should be able to design, "unencumbered by ethical constraints," according to Gunn and Vesilind (1990).

The fact still remains, nonetheless, that professionals are multidimensional. They apply a systematic body of acquired knowledge and specific skills not easily standardized. In this respect they offer to society a service that the lay person cannot offer. Their decisions have the potential to affect the lives of those they serve significantly. Therefore,

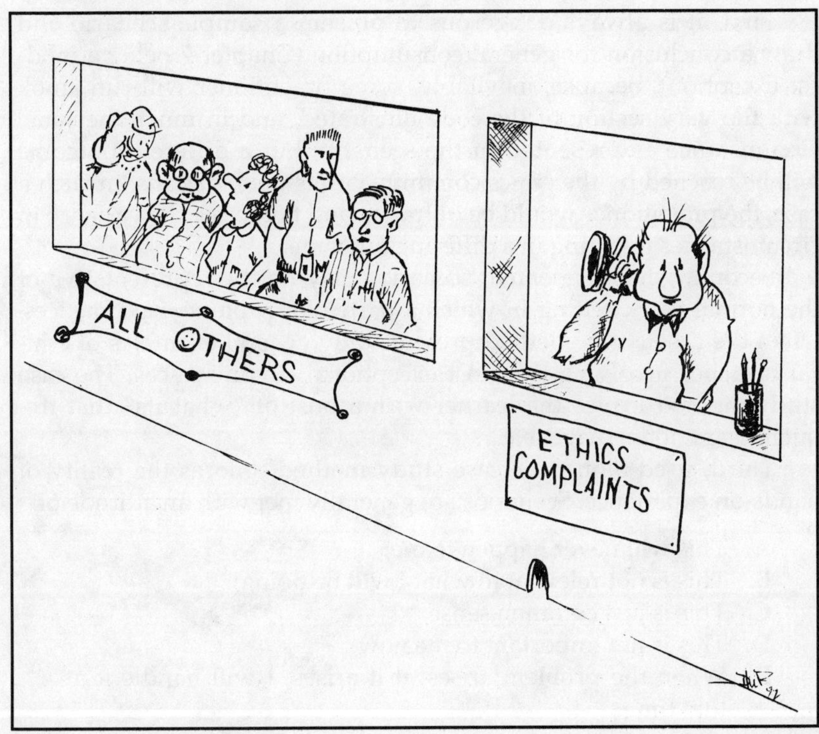

their conduct must deserve a high level of public trust. There is no room for even the appearance of impropriety. There is much room for ethical conduct.

In focusing attention on the need for schooling in professional ethics the emphasis must be directed toward methods that develop sensitivity toward ethical thinking to **avoid** problems—not to finding an ethical solution to problems once they have emerged. Traditional teaching methods may be quite unsuitable for achieving this goal. Professors may not be able to **teach** ethics. New approaches may be necessary, but such a stumbling block does not detract from the need to instill professional ethics early in the training of practitioners (Waggoner, 1990).

One of the common approaches to developing an understanding of ethics is the **case study** method. It is the one used in this book, for example, in an attempt to provide a path for procedural guidelines in specific instances of apparent ethical misconduct. Although the method should not be underestimated, it is not without limitations and even dangers.

First, it is always dangerous to present a sample scenario and draw a conclusion for general consumption (Chapter 7 being a modest exception), because, inevitably, some practitioner will run amok with the very section of the code illustrated, and in much the same circumstance as presented in the scenario, but a different outcome will be reached by the ethics committee in its deliberations. In such a case, the practitioner would be outraged and fail to see the variance in circumstances resulting in a differing outcome.

Second, when presented, scenarios may not be representative of the normal work setting in which a particular professional practices. Often the case study method presents only general examples of ethical breaches involving the most exceptional circumstances. The case study method leaves the learner with a host of "what ifs" that frequently are not manageable.

Third, used alone, the case study method ignores the reality of hands-on experience. Scenarios are generally met with an attitude of:

A. This will never happen to me;
B. This is not relevant to what I will be doing;
C. This is just common sense;
D. This is not important to me now;
E. When the problem arises, if it arises, I will handle it at that time.

Most people, generally speaking, will follow the ethical principles set forth in their professional codes of ethics. Those in training, the preprofessionals, can also be expected to do the right thing. At least in the beginning they will listen to the professor and absorb what the teacher says is the "best" approach to a problem of ethics. That, of course, is fine until the code of ethics comes into conflict with the person's own value system. Then a different set of criteria emerge.

One of the values of including the gift scenario in this text, despite the acknowledged limitations of the case study approach, is to have readers say to themselves that the value of the gift or the circumstances under which it was offered, coupled with the short- and long-range consequences of accepting (or rejecting) it, and the number of persons affected by the acceptance (or rejection) of the gift make acceptance imprudent, questionably ethical, definitely unethical, morally wrong, illegal, or potentially troublesome. If this went through your mind as you read that particular scenario, good! If not, read it again. (Look again at the other scenarios as well.)

Professionals have a responsibility to think about ethics and issues relevant to ethics. These issues might be those involved with social ethics, business ethics, bioethics, professional ethics, and/or the ethics of abortion/right to life, capital punishment, homelessness, civil rights, gay rights, and on and on. There is an obligation that goes with the territory of every profession to take charge of the ethical conduct and climate under which that profession is delivered to the public. Everything points toward an increase in the demand for ethical accountability among the professions. The professions must respond effectively while they are still in control of their destiny.

THE ETHICS PAINS OF AUDIOLOGY

Audiology, more so than speech-language pathology, is passing through a very trying period in its growth. This is largely the case because today audiology dispenses, that is *sells* an item of merchandise as part of the service it provides to the hearing impaired. From before the 1950s until late into the 1980s, this was not allowed by the association's code of ethics. Instead, audiologists who functioned in the private sector, that is, nonmilitary, nongovernment programs, evaluated patients, selected hearing aid amplification, and then referred the patient to a commercial seller of hearing aids who sold the instrument as recommended by the audiologist—and kept the profit.

There was not much opportunity for a conflict of interest situation in those times, although occasionally a local vendor "repaid" for a referral with a box of cashews, a bottle of wine, or a Christmas ham. No one gave much attention to it because it didn't seem to make a lot of difference. Audiologists kept those who sold hearing aids at arm's length and that seemed to be an acceptable distance to both parties.

For the seller of hearings aids the process was a mixed blessing. The good news was that a professional referral from an audiologist represented an easy sale. The bad news was that the seller was stuck with whatever fitting or more accurately, perhaps, *misfitting* problems the audiologist happened to create. Most unfortunate for the audiologist was that the consumer identified with the seller rather than the audiologist and returned there for future care. The ethics of the entire process were never questioned, although it seemed strange for an audiologist to refer a referral to yet another party.

A few audiologists who actually sold hearing aids in partial attempt to retain professional control and thereby provide quality service to the consumer were expelled from the professional association for a violation of the code that did not permit audiologists to participate in the actual sale of an instrument. As audiology became more of an independent discipline, however, and moved into the private sector, the habits of practice changed, too.

In the 1970s audiologists began to dispense hearing devices as part of their service. The Code of Ethics of the association still didn't permit it, but most practitioners were doing it anyway. Finally the code was revised to be in line with actual practice and render the sale of hearing aids by audiologists as an ethical practice. The act of dispensing the instrument as one part of the total rehabilitative management of hearing-impaired patients has both positive and negative vibrations.

The good side of the issue is that by actually dispensing the recommended prosthesis to the user, the audiologist maintains high control over the rehabilitative management of the person. One crucial step in enhancing auditory capability, that of providing amplification, remains with the audiologist who has recommended it.

The bad side is that the process smacks of a built-in conflict of interest. Such a conflict may very well not be there, but it appears to exist, and that's too bad, because the procedure is a method of providing hearing aids to people who require them through a much improved process compared to the officially supported standard prior to 1991.

Whether the move was a good one or not, will only be shown by time. Several questions are raised in regard to the consumer, however:

1. How is the consumer protected against conflict of interest surrounding the audiologist who now stands to benefit financially from the sale of the product prescribed? How is the audiologist shielded from the apparent *appearance* of conflict surrounding the recommendation and sale of products?
2. What is the difference between the commercial seller of hearing aids (licensed as a vendor) and an audiologist hearing aid dispenser (also licensed as vendor) in the eyes of the consumer?
3. Should consumers be told of the special discount arrangements that accompany the audiologist's purchases?

There is no doubt that the day a professional, any professional, requested a fee for services, economics and conflict of interest entered the arena. It is fair for laymen to point to professional fees and presume the prescription of a professional's services/products by the practitioner is a means of maintaining the prescriber's own income.

Socrates in his dialogue with Thrasymachus, as described in Plato's *Republic*, admitted that physicians were engaged in two "arts": the art of medicine with its end the health of the patient and the art of making money with its end the self-interest of the physician. For an even more enlightening and modern version of the fee dilemma, no one has more tellingly exposed the inevitability of a certain amount of conflict of interest in every professional's work, than George Bernard Shaw (1965).

Beneficence

The *de facto* conflict of interest associated with professional fees in return for services is virtually impossible to eliminate, given that professionals must earn a living to support families and have access to the same material goods as others. What mitigates the obvious conflict, though, is the professional's ethical commitment to the patient's good. Another way to refer to the patient's good is to call it the principle of beneficence.

Beneficence has always implied rather clearly some degree of effacement of a professional's self-interest in favor of the interest of the patient. For centuries, for example, physicians have treated patients who could not pay, have exposed themselves to contagious disease or physical harm in responding to all requests for care simply out of commitments to serve the good of the patient. This effacement of self-interest is, in fact, the very point that distinguishes a true profession from a business trade or craft. It is the expectation that professionals will, to an overwhelming extent, practice a generous degree of effacement justifying the trust that individuals and society place in them.

Beneficence, as a matter of fact, provides an accepted and professional underpinning for an attractive model of health care with deep ethics roots. There are other models, of course, but the beneficence model is easily understood and incorporates the good parts of all the others. It is especially appropriate to preservation of professional dominance in the fields of audiology and speech-language pathology.

ETHICS AND MODELS OF HEALTH CARE

Childress and Siegler (1984) examine how different systems of metaphors and models of health care are responsible for conditioning the way practitioners view their provider roles and their moral principles. Different models sometimes lead to competing views about the moral principles involved in health care and even in the virtues exhibited by those who practice in the various branches of the professions. The practice attitude of any professional can be described by any of the following models. Beneficence is, however, the paradigm that offers the most hope for preserving the professions.

The Business Relation Model

In the business relation model health care is viewed as a commodity, and purchasing health care is a transaction not too different from buying an automobile, a house, or a refrigerator. The business relation model is often used by hospital administrators, health planners, and economists who view health services as product lines to be evaluated by their economic viability, market attractiveness, and, for that matter, income-producing capabilities. When local television commercials speak to the availability and convenience of reconstructive plastic surgery to make you feel better about yourself, the chances are that the practice advertised is driven by the business relation model.

In some professions private practice health care becomes a commodity to be bought and sold in the marketplace. Some commodities sell better than others—coronary artery bypass surgery, for example, is a good seller. Some sell well but do not pay well—cochlear implant surgery and tune-up, for instance. In some practices the purchaser is goaded into buying at the best price. Everyone is happy when the purchaser pays all charges on time, is a repeat customer, follows advice and instructions, and refers other people to the same source for purchases—or so it seems.

The ethical obligations of the provider in the business model are to provide a good "product" and stand behind it. The product can be strictly service, or clearly product such as eyeglasses, hearing aids, or an electrolarynx. The provider can charge whatever the traffic will bear, and the consumer will pay whatever the care or product is considered worth. For the purchasing patient the guiding principle is caveat emptor; for the caregiver, primacy goes to providing a good service (product), not only because it is morally owed to the patient, but because it is good business to be known for good service.

The ethical obligations of the business model are merely the ethics of good business and good consumerism. To make certain that the relationship between the buyer and the seller doesn't go awry, however, the obligations of the provider and the recipient to each other, in addition to being based in ethics, have legal aspects, and transactions can be tested in court.

The Contractual Relation Model

The contractual relation model has all the characteristics of the business model, but requirements of the transacting parties are explicit. The model grows in popularity daily, because so many people wish to protect themselves from the paternalism and apparent economic self-interest of medical practitioners. It becomes more attractive, too, because of the various gatekeeping roles required of medical practitioners.

This model treats both caregiver and consumer as equal partners in a commodity transaction, but seeks to limit the region of trust between practitioner and consumer. The contractual model mitigates somewhat the principle of caveat emptor, but it generates the same ethical requirements. These are largely those based in law rather than morality. It interprets justice, truth-telling, promise-keeping, nonmaleficence, and beneficence as legal terms rather than as trust in the virtue of the participants in the transaction. In other words, it is a contract executed for certain items under specified conditions for a given number of people and for a given dollar amount. It might be the sort of model followed by a speech-language pathology practice in negotiating to manage the speech problems of children in a private school, for example. Who does what to whom under what circumstances and in exchange for what items of value are specified and agreed to by the parties involved. Trust is bound in the terms of the contract.

Subscribing to a health maintenance organization (HMO) health care plan is essentially a contractual health services model. The subscriber buys in for a specified dollar amount and the HMO agrees to meet the policy holder's needs within certain boundaries. Recall the positive gatekeeping described in an earlier chapter and ponder how that philosophy shapes the contract relation model.

The strongest criticism of the contract relation model is in the assumption that the contracting parties are truly equal. It is difficult to envision someone who is ill, in need of help, worried, and so on as equal in the face of, say, a physician's knowledge and skill. Being denied service because the event was not covered in a contract minimizes the faith and trust traditionally afforded to professional providers of health care by reducing give-and-take to contractual terms.

Professional ethics are at risk in the contract model. That is not to state categorically that a violation of professional ethics is bound to occur among practitioners engaged in providing services under a contract model. It is, however, to suggest that strong motivations exist in the model that do not mesh comfortably with the traditional principles of professions.

The Covenant Model

The covenant model grounds the relationship between caregiver and consumer in the sacred, with rich connotations of trust and obligation. It is the opposite of the concept of a legal contract or a commodity transaction. The covenant model is steeped in the concepts of social justice, theories of social obligation, and views of patient autonomy. It seeks to allow the recipient of care to contribute to that care and even to refuse care. The covenant model is applied well in matters of bioethics.

The covenant model operates defensibly in many institutional settings where debate among interested parties is not only accepted, but expected. The ethics of giver and receiver in the covenant model are solid because the system allows for an acceptance of the wishes of both parties in satisfying needs. If there is criticism to be levied, it is that a great deal of philosophizing takes place in the covenant model. It is more applicable to institutions than private practice activities.

The Preventive Model

The preventive model rejects legal contracts, covenants, or other bonding mechanisms. In the preventive model, health care is not considered as a relationship between giver and receiver at all. Instead caregivers become social engineers and engineer society to protect as many "healths" as possible by establishing social policies for a healthy population. As examples, the preventive model encourages walking, jogging, aerobics, brushing teeth, wearing sunscreen, establishing wellness programs, and so on. It is aimed at prevention, and if it were to be 100% successful, there would be no need for any other model.

The issue appears to be that it is far better to prevent the need for health care than to seek economical, ethical, efficient ways to provide for those who are ill. The preventive concept is found extensively outside the United States of America. The ethics of the system are less obvious or open to discussion than the other models.

The Beneficent Model

The beneficent model of health care incorporates the best points of all the others without having to include the failings. In this model the caregiver and the patient are joined by the bond of a particular kind of need. The need, of course, is for healing, and it makes little difference what that healing may be or whether, for that matter, it be the need for advice, guidance, support counseling, and so forth.

The caregiver is the one who responds to the need of the care seeker and makes right (correct) and good (moral) judgments with, and on behalf of, the one in need. Health care, then, is a negotiable good in the beneficent model. It is not an absolute and overriding value. It does not have a fixed cost to be negotiated by the parties involved. It is a simple pattern of two needs being mutually satisfied; the need of the provider to give care is met by the person whose need to receive care is then satisfied by the giver.

In this model the patient suffers a need that cannot be overcome without help from another who is trained and credentialed to provide relief for the need. The patient is dependent on another human being who *professes* to be able to help, once again, contrasting the professional with the tradesman.

The bond of need creates an obligation in the professional to act on behalf of the patient. The health professions are ordained by society primarily for this purpose and *not* for entrepreneurship. It is *that* recognition motivating all the fuss over ethics. The patient needs and trusts the caregiver.

When evidence begins to emerge that an erosion in that trust is occurring, it's time to make an even greater fuss over ethics.

10

The End or
the Beginning?

Never bunt on third strike.   (My father)

Benevolence in health care, *wishing* for the patient's good, and beneficence, *doing* the patient's good arise from several sources. For example, both wishing and doing good may arise from respect for the inherent rights of other people, from recognition of the duties and obligations of a practiced profession, by just being a person who out of habit desires the right thing or even being the one who always does the good thing. The ethics of today seem to place the emphasis on the respect for rights and duties. But, in the long run it is the caregiver's character, or *virtues* that provides the final guarantee that the health care consumer's good will be respected. The guarantees of rights-and-duty-based ethics, doing good, are dependent on the character of the professional caregiver, however, and in some intricate way related to virtue-based ethics, wishing good, to provide maximal protection of all dimensions of what professionals do to enhance the patient's good. It is difficult, if not downright impossible, to separate the *doing* from the *wishing* good, but somehow it seems better to *do* than to merely *wish*. The old expression that "it's the thought that counts" does not fit well in the ethics of doing good in providing health care.

It is also difficult to forecast whether the erosion in ethics apparent in most walks of life at the end of this century describes the denouement of an era of virtue for everybody and is a harbinger of what is to come in the decades ahead, or rather represents a general moral catharsis required before a rebuilding of faith in a system girded by other than self-interest.

Certainly awareness of professional ethics is sensitized by the persistent changes in behavior, the discovery of relationships between business and profession heretofore unrecognized, and the adjustments made by some professions to regain trust. The hope is that awareness will bring improvement, restoration of virtues, and soundness of ethic to the professions. The result is by no means guaranteed, however, although the roots of virtues apparently run long and deep.

ONE CONCEPT OF VIRTUE

The virtues have always hovered over most theories of morals. Virtues give credibility to human life and assure that life will be something more than a catalog of rights, duties, and rules. Virtue adds that extra cubit elevating ethics out of legalisms and into the higher reaches of moral sensitivity.

As Pellegrino (1988) points out, however, virtue-based ethics is a dubious enterprise. With the mere wishing of good there no longer is a prior vantage point from which to judge what is right and good. Virtue becomes confused with the conformity to the conventions of social adjustment and institutional life. The accolades accrue to those who go along with the trends and get ahead, many times without knowing what the right and the good may mean or whether right and good were even done. The attitude is essentially, "I'm okay because I say I am, therefore you're okay because I say you are."

These uncertainties, perhaps better described as unprovables, force a reliance on ethical systems built on *specific* rights, duties, and the application of principles and rules. The very concreteness of such systems seems to promise protection against capricious and anti-ethical interpretations of vice and virtue. But even that concreteness turns to illusion when an attempt is made to agree on what is the right and good thing to do in a certain professional situation. Tangential considerations weaken the forces of virtue and at times strengthen the trends of vice. There are many examples presented in this book.

Despite an apparent erosion of at least the virtue concept of ethics, virtue remains an inescapable reality in moral transactions of nearly every type. There clearly are people who can be trusted to temper self-interest, to be honest, truthful, faithful, and just, even in the face of evil. Most people fit that description. Sadly, there are others who cannot be trusted to habitually act well in the most unpressured of circumstances. We may not be virtuous ourselves, yet we can recognize virtue in others. As Marcus Aurelius (Oates 1957) said, "No thing delights as much as examples of the virtues when they are exhibited in the morals of those who live with us and present themselves in abundance as far as possible."

Truth to be known, the virtues are once more gaining a toe-hold in the resurgence of interest in virtue-based ethics. Much of what has preceded in this book is testimony, and it is as though the end had turned once again toward the beginning to start anew. In the main, the resurgence is based in a re-examination, clarification, and refurbishment of the classical-medieval concept of virtue (Kenny, 1978; Wallace, 1978). The reappraisal is not an abnegation of rights-and-duty-based ethics, but rather a recognition that moral effectiveness still turns on the disposition and character traits of collegial men and women. Running counter is the madness of health care rationing that spills its negative traits on the professions, forcing a rethinking, perhaps requiring a change in philosophy. The rationing of health care, positive and negative gate-keeping models of care delivery, and the burgeoning business opportunities open to the professions provide examples.

The vulnerability and dependency of the sick person force a trust not just in rights, but in the *kind* of person the caregiver is as well. In the search for health care, when people are perhaps most exploitable, they seek to depend on the kind of person who will do the right thing because the provider cannot really do otherwise. How stalwart can the ethics of a profession be expected to be? Is that even a fair question, or should the question instead be directed at the need for professional ethics at all, especially in the turbulent waters of skyrocketing health care costs? The trust given to the professions is at stake. The assumption is that most professions want trust preserved as the foundation of their endeavor. Some may not care. But if they do not, they cannot last as professions.

The variability with which this trust is honored and, at times, its outright violation account for the unfortunate present decline in the moral credibility of many professions. The situation accounts, too, for the trend of patients asserting rights more forcefully in contractual instead of to covenantal models of patient–caregiver relationships. Consider the HMO model where all care is directed by a primary-care physician. Does this represent the initial step toward national health insurance, and if so, what will be the imprint it will leave on the ethics of a profession? And what of the virtues?

TWO KINDS OF VIRTUE

Virtue is of two kinds: intellectual and moral. Intellectual virtue requires both experience and time and owes its birth and growth to teaching.

Moral virtue is the result of habit. Virtue, then, is a state of character, not simply a passion or a culture. It is that state of character that defines a people as good and that makes them do their own work well. States of character, nevertheless, must be in accord with the "right rule." Hence, the intellectual virtues play a significant part in making a person virtuous.

In the past several years the classical concept of virtue has been re-examined by a growing number of moral philosophers. They have underscored such things as the difference in meanings of the words *arete* in Greek, *virtutes* in Latin, and *virtue* in English (although all three mean the same thing); the distinctions between virtues and skills; the difficulty in defining words such as disposition and habit; the relationship between virtue, value, and concepts of good and their relationship with duties, rights, and obligations. It is a way of describing the ethics of a situation. Perhaps, too, it is an exercise in futility. Perhaps not.

Some people dispense with further discussion of what virtue is by saying of virtue what has been said of pornography, "I can't define it, but I know it when I see it." The assumption is that even though the doer is unable to tell someone what a wrongful act is, they are able to recognize one and therefore would not actually commit such an act. That view of virtue is not sufficient in today's professions and in many marketplaces, but virtuous traits are.

VIRTUOUS TRAITS

Virtue implies a character trait, an internal disposition to seek moral perfection, to live one's life in accord with moral law, and to achieve a balance between noble intention and just action. That's the blueprint. Perhaps one can liken the virtuous person to the good golfer. When one refers to a good golfer one is describing someone whose eyes, muscles, and nerves have been so trained to a fine degree by making innumerable good shots that the aspects can be relied on to correctly coordinate over and over and over. The person's body has a certain tone that is present even when the person is not in contest play. In the same way, a person who perseveres in doing things in a just way lives in the end with a recognizable quality of character. It is in the long haul *that* quality of character rather than particular actions taken that is meant when one speaks of virtue.

The virtuous person is, then, someone who will act habitually in a good way—courageously, honestly, justly, wisely, and so on. The virtuous person is committed to *being* a good person and to the pursuit of perfection in private, professional, and community life. The virtuous person will act well even when there is no one to applaud, simply because to act otherwise is a violation of what it is to be a good human being.

No civilized society could endure without a certain number of citizens committed to this concept of virtue. Without such persons, no system of ethics would succeed either, and no system of professional ethics could transcend the dangers of self-interest. That is the reason why, even while rights, duties, and obligations may be emphasized, the aura of virtue has hung so persistently over every system of ethics since Hippocrates.

One could easily ask whether we are, in fact, talking about the end or the beginning here, or for that matter whether virtues are even peculiar to professions. Similarly, one could wonder whether some virtues are more applicable to professions than elsewhere in human life? How do professional skills differ from virtue?

There is perhaps a better chance of coming closer to the relationships of virtue to clinical or professional actions if one looks to the more immediate ends of pure health care encounters. The "good" the patient seeks of health care, for example, is to be made well—to be restored to his or her prior or, perhaps, even better state of function, to be made whole again. If this is cannot be, the patient expects to be helped to deal with the pain, suffering, dying, or limitation that the illness may entail. The immediate end of health care is not merely a technically proficient performance, but the use of that performance to attain a good end, the good of the patient—"above all, do no harm."

While virtue may be necessary to obtain the good intrinsic to, say, medicine as a practice, values exist independently of medicine and can be applied to nearly any professional endeavor. They are necessary to the practice of a good life, no matter in what activities that life may express itself.

Professionalism calls forth benevolence, beneficence, truthfulness, more fidelity than physical courage, for instance, although that could be debated if one were to stand with the medic who ministers to soldiers on the battlefield. But that is not the issue here.

A person can cultivate technical professional skills to a superlative degree for reasons other than the good of the patient—personal pride, profit, prestige, power, aggrandizement. Such a practitioner can make technically correct decisions and perform skillfully, but would not be considered virtuous and could not be depended on to act against self-interest for the good of the patient.

In the virtuous caregiver, for instance, the explicit fulfillment of rights and duties is an overt expression of an inner disposition to do the right and the good. One is, then, virtuous not only because one has conformed to the letter of the law, but because that is what a good person does. Ethics starts with one's commitment to be a certain kind of person and then approaches the clinical quandaries, value conflicts, and patient interests as a good person ought. Ethics, by written code, assures insofar as possible, that the *good person* attitude is sustained, and that it is open, obvious, and available to the consumer. If one is a good person (has the virtue), a written code of ethical behavior is not a bothersome document. It is when one tends to scale the periphery of virtue that the written code of conduct becomes an annoyance.

The professions that deal with the more sensitive facets and nuances of a care seeker's background must exercise virtue more diligently than technique-oriented specialists. The narrower the specialty the more easily the consumer's good can be safeguarded by rules of ethics; the broader the specialty, the more significant are the practitioner's character traits. In that analogy, then, one might say that the practice of internal medicine, or perhaps speech-language pathology, requires greater attention to the character traits of the practitioner than is the case with the practice of otolaryngology, or audiology, or optometry. No branch of medicine or any profession, for that matter, can be carried on without dedication to some of the virtue. Most professionals do more than their solely self-interest share of attending to the welfare of the person served.

Regrettably, however, people do compartmentalize their lives. Professionals can practice properly, yet be guilty of vice in their personal lives. Others pay little attention to the character of their relationships with those to whom owe special consideration—children, spouse, and so on. There are, for example, many instances of physicians who seek the good for their patients and neglect obligations to their family. Such a person could not be called a virtuous physician. One could not be secure in, or trust, such a person's disposition to act in a right and good way—even in medicine. One of the essential aspects of virtue is balancing conflicting obligations judiciously. It is one of the more difficult features. It is again the matter of jurisdiction.

LIMITATIONS OF VIRTUE-BASED ETHICS

It is only proper to note that there are some logical difficulties with virtue-based ethics. For one thing, there is no full agreement as to a definition of *virtue*. There are synonyms and antonyms, but no widely accepted definition. For another, there is some circular thought to the assertion that virtue is what the good people do by habit, and at the same time asserting that one becomes virtuous by always doing good.

Virtue and good are defined in terms of each other, and that may not be an accurate starting point. It becomes particularly limiting if there is no agreement on the concrete principles to specify, for example, in the development of a code of ethics. In light of these limitations, a virtue-based ethics system is difficult to defend as the sole basis of normative judgments.

Having pointed that out it should also be seen that these same deficiencies are evident in rights-and-duty-based ethics. The good of the patient cannot be protected by rights and duties alone. Some degree of supererogation is vital in the relationship between those in need of health care and those who profess to provide it.

Most professional ethics codes are a blend of virtue and duty. The Oath of Hippocrates, as an example, imposes certain duties, such as protection of privacy, avoiding performance of abortion, and not harming the patient. Additionally, however, the Hippocratic physician also pledges to "guard his life and his art." This is an exhortation to be a good person and a virtuous practitioner in order to serve in an ethically responsible way. Likewise, the first century writer Scribonius Largus (Pellegrino & Thomasma, 1988) made compassion a virtue essential to the professions.

Recall from an earlier chapter that the 1980 version of the AMA Principles of Medical Ethics intermingles duties, rights, and virtue. The document refers to standards of conduct, essentials of honorable behavior, dealing honestly with patients and colleagues, etc. Those who cynically deny any virtue by physicians may very well interpret those standards as the final remnants of a fading tradition of altruistic benevolence. At the very least, nonetheless, the principles attest to the recognition that the good of the patient cannot be assured by rights and duties alone. We all know that.

ASCENDING VIRTUE SYSTEM

It is reasonable to state that all professional ethics codes are constructed of a three-tiered system of obligations based on the special role of professionals in society. In ascending order of ethical sensitivity these are (1) observance of the laws of the land, (2) observance of human rights and fulfillment of duties, and (3) the practice of virtue.

The second level is the ethics of rights and duties beyond those defined by the law. At this level, benevolence and beneficence take on more than just legal meanings. The ideal of service, of responsiveness to the needs and trust of those who seek care, along with varying degrees of compassion, kindliness, honesty are included in this level. Just how these principles are invoked and how conflicts among them are resolved in the patient's best interest are topics of widely swinging interpretations.

But virtue-based ethics goes even beyond these two levels. Virtue ethics expands the notions of benevolence, beneficence, compassion, fidelity, right, good, and all the rest far beyond what strict duty might require. It calls for standards of ethical performance that exceed those in the rest of society (Reeder, 1982). At each of the levels, there are dangers from overzealous observance, just as there are perils from paltry attention to the social rules of professional practice.

Legalistic ethics systems tend toward minimal ethics, a thin definition of benevolence and beneficence, and a contract-minded relationship between caregiver and recipient. Rights- and duty-based ethics may be overly weighted to rule worship and a stringent compliance with the letter of the ethics rules to the exclusion of the modifications and nuances the spirit of those principles implies. A virtue-based ethic can easily lapse into self-righteous professionalism or unwelcome overinvolvement in the personal life of the practitioner as well as the patient.

Professional ethics based in virtue distinguishes itself less by the avoidance of immoral practices than by the avoidance of practices at the margin of moral respectability. It is the decay of ethics at each of these levels that has professions concerned because the temptations are great and may even become greater.

ALTRUISM PITTED AGAINST SELF-INTEREST

Professionals are confronted in today's morally relaxed climate with a countless number of practices pitting altruism against self-interest. Most are not allowed or, at the very least, are defined as immoral in a rigid rights- and duty-based ethic. They are also inconsistent with the higher levels of moral sensitivity that a virtue based ethic demands.

The practices can be grouped into four categories:

A. Making a profit from the illness or abnormality of others;
B. Limiting the concept of service for personal convenience;
C. Taking a proprietary attitude with regard to professional knowledge;
D. Placing loyalty to the profession above loyalty to those served.

For physicians such things as investment in and ownership of for-profit hospitals, hospital chains, nursing homes, dialysis clinics, diagnostic centers, (re)habilitation facilities; tie-in arrangements with X-ray or laboratory services; escalation of fees for repetitive, high-volume procedures; dispensing of products readily available in the marketplace are squarely in category A. For audiologists and speech-language pathologists investment in or ownership of business models that provide practitioners for rent to facilities throughout the country might similarly fit into category A.

The second type of morally questionable practice would include income-based availability and accessibility of professional practitioners in a given specialty; the diffusion of responsibility to patients in professional group practices; the delegation of services to an unsupervised practitioner-in-training without full knowledge and consent of the consumer of those services; overindulgence in self-development; overreferral within a group are examples of category B. Under certain circumstances, audiologists and speech-language pathologists who employ trainee-level staff, including CFY candidates, might be described under certain circumstances as fitting into category B.

The third category might include "selling one's services" for whatever the market will bear; patenting new procedures or keeping processes secret from colleagues; becoming a professional court witness as a primary means of self-support. These practices are clearly proprietary and place the doer in category C.

The final category might include making referrals on the basis of friendship or reciprocity rather than skill; resisting consultations and second opinions; placing the interest of the referral source above the interest of the patient; looking the other way in the face of incompetence or dishonesty in professional colleagues.

These and other practices go on and are even encouraged in some professions in today's attitude of competition. None can be rationalized in virtue-based ethics. A virtue-based ethics simply does not fluctuate with what the dominant social mores will tolerate. A virtue-based ethics is inherently elitist because it interprets benevolence, beneficence, and responsibility in a way that addresses the central paradox in most professions by reducing self-interest and enhancing altruism.

It is entirely possible that society in the short run will choose to ignore all of the attributes of ethics and the professions and will choose other values over health. Society may in fact envision health care in the 21st century as little more than a commodity or service like any other business. And like any business, the Golden Rule may be eventually a perfectly adequate ethic for professions to adopt. Physicians will indeed become the gatekeepers of health care, and the cornerstones of professional ethics—beneficence, patient autonomy, and justice—would then give way to social good and economic need. But that level of protective consumerism is not yet here.

Neither the professions nor the public can have it both ways: On the one hand the professional cannot be mandated to serve the interest of the consumer, and on the other be expected to be the instrument of social policy as well as an advocate of the consumer of health services.

ANOTHER VIEW

It is equally possible that the standards of care to which professionals are currently held will be downgraded to accommodate the pressures of society and the kinds of decisions which will then be required. When that happens, however, the legal profession will become a partner in health care, wanted or not. Everyone will need protection from the presumption that standards of care can be reduced without sacrifice to the safety of the consumer. The problem is that the assumption that the consumer of health care will accept less if the cost is less is risky. When it comes to health care, very few people are willing to compromise their own safety. The public will undoubtedly continue to demand professionalism, but it will be more difficult to provide. The public will offer its trust, but the offer will have few takers.

The differences between present and proposed standards of health care are not trivial. The important issue looming as a deterrent to the preservation of ethics is whether a reduction in the quality of care (sure to go beyond simply eliminating the frills and unnecessaries) would free professional practitioners from their ethical obligations; and further questions the viable future of ethics codes supported by the professions.

One of the most common practices in which prepayment health care or for-profit plans affect the quality of care presented to the recipient is referred to as "economic transfer." When a patient presents for admission to a hospital, for instance, as in the case of Nancy Ellen Jobes[1], insurance coverage and ability to pay are assessed along with the medical condition. When patients are judged to be an economic risk they are transferred to a publicly supported institution. Of course, the transferring physician does not evaluate this obligation in a willy-nilly manner. Patients are assumed stable, and transfer is judged not to be a medical endangerment. Nonetheless, patients have suffered damage, physically and emotionally, as a result of this practice. Is it reasonable to presume that the economics of health care will affect the ethics of audiology and speech-language services? Maybe.

But once again, the impact that the economic transfer has on the ethics of the practitioner seems indefensible. The conflict of interest is obvious and explicit in situations such as this. Moral responsibility

---

[1] *In the matter of Nancy Ellen Jobes,* Superior Court of N. J. Chancery Division, Morris County, docket no. C-4971-85E, April 23, 1986.

has shifted and has become diluted; once more the paradox of an economic and market system exploits the self-interest of the practitioner. The public's expectation is deluded.

Recognition of the ethical dilemmas created by the growing national belief that health care rationing in order to provide care for everyone is inevitable. The impact on the nature of professional ethics is, or at least soon will be, apparent. These are matters of wide public, as well as professional concern. More change may take place in professional ethics in the next decade than in the 2,500-year history of medical ethics. For medicine it is the post-Hippocratic era. For the professions as a whole it is an era of doubt as to whether any can exist with a common set of principles deserving the public trust. The voting is not over.

Perhaps this book will have a positive effect in producing a better understanding of the ethics of a profession. The author has informed the reader about professional ethics and has made a case for its preservation. The underlying thread throughout the book is the belief that the essence of a profession lies in its public commitment to act in certain ways necessary to its role in society. Intertwined in that fundamental tenet is the further belief that a true profession is distinguished from all other human endeavors by its commitment to a higher degree of altruism and finally in the belief that the obligations of all health professionals are underpinned by the nature of the abnormalities that they manage, by the faithfulness of their promise to help, and by the enormous power of their knowledge and skill.

Perhaps with a better understanding of professional ethics, whether those ethics be interpreted as virtue-based, or rights- and duty-based a reconstruction of the ethics foundation that undergirds all professions can be begin. Perhaps, too, even a greater degree of progress can be made by heeding Shakespeare's advice in Hamlet:

> "Assume the virtue if you have it not. . . . For use almost can change the stamp of nature."

References

American Academy of Audiology. (1991). *Code of ethics*. Houston: American Academy of Audiology.

American College of Physicians, Ad hoc Committee on Medical Ethics. (1984). *American College of Physicians Manual, 101*, 129–137.

American Medical Association. (1848). Code of medical ethics: Adopted by the American Medical Association at Philadelphia, May 1847, and by the New York Academy of Medicine in October, 1847. New York: H. Ludwig.

American Medical Association v. FTC, 638 F. 2d 443, 447 (2d Cir. 1980).

American Medical Association. (1981). *Current opinions of the Judicial Council of the American Medical Association*. Chicago: American Medical Association.

American Medical Association. (1984). *Current opinions of the Judicial Council of the American Medical Association: Including the Principles of Medical Ethics and Rules of the Judicial Council*. Chicago: American Medical Association.

American Medical Association. (1986). *Current opinions of the council on ethical and judicial affairs*. Section 8.06. Chicago: American Medical Association.

American Medical Association. (August, 1988). *Medical technology innovation: Pre-requisite to quality health care* (White Paper). Chicago: American Medical Association.

American Medical Association. (1991). *Report of the council on ethical and judicial affairs*. Chicago: American Medical Association.

American Nurses' Association, Committee on Ethics. (1979). *Ethics in nursing: References and resources*. Kansas City: American Nurses' Association.

American Optometric Association. (1976). *Code of ethics and standards of practice*. St. Louis: American Optometric Association.

American Optometric Association v. FTC, 626 F. 2d 896 D.C. Cir. (1980).

American Society of Hospital Pharmacists. (1992). ASHP guidelines on pharmacists' relationships with industry. *American Journal of Hospital Pharmacists, 49*.

American Speech-Language-Hearing Association. (1991). *Code of ethics* (rev. 1991). Rockville, MD: American Speech-Language-Hearing Association.

American Speech-Language-Hearing Association. (1992). *Code of ethics* (rev. 1992). Rockville, MD: American Speech-Language-Hearing Association.

Aurelius, M. (1957). "Meditations", VI, 48, in W. J.Oates, Ed., *The stoic and epicurean philosophers*. New York: Modern Library.

Avorn, J. (1982). The influence of marketing on drug utilization. *American Journal of Medicine, 73,* 4–8.

Bleich, J. (1979). The obligation to heal in the Judaic tradition: A comparative analysis. In F. Rosner & J. Bleich (Eds.), *Jewish Bioethics* (pp. 1–44). New York: Sanhedrin Press.

Blumenthal, D. (1986). University-industry research relationships in biotechnology: Implications for the university. *Science, 232,* 1361–1366.

British Medical Association. (1984). *The handbook of medical ethics.* Luton and London: Leagrave Press.

Bush v. Dake, No. 86-25767 NM (Michigan Cir. Ct. 1988).

California Association of Psychology Providers v. Rank, 793 2d 2, (Cal. 1990).

Catlin, R., Bradbury, R. C., & Catlin, R.J.O. (1983). Primary care gatekeepers in HMOs. *The Journal of Family Practice, 17,* 673–678.

Childress, J., & Siegler, M. (1984). Metaphors and models of doctor-patient relationships: Their implications for autonomy, *Theoretical Medicine, 5,* 17–36.

Corbet v. D'Allesandro, 487 So. 2d 386 (Va. App. 1985).

Culliton, B.J. (1988). Conflict of interest eyed at Harvard. *Science, 242,* 1497–1501.

Curran, J., & Harford, E. (1991, November-December). Point: Counterpoint, *Audiology Today, 3,* 6.

Edelstein, L. (1967). The Hippocratic oath: Text, translation, interpretation. In O. Temkin & L. Temkin (Eds.), *Ancient medicine: Selected Papers of Ludwig Edelstein* (C.L. Temkin, trans.), (pp.3–64). Baltimore: Johns Hopkins Press.

Eisenberg, J.M. (1985). The internist as gatekeeper. *Annals of Internal Medicine. 102,* 4, 537–543.

Etziony, M. B. (1973). *The physician's creed: An anthology of medical prayers, oaths, and codes of ethics written and recited by medical practitioners through the ages.* Springfield, IL: Charles Thomas.

Federal Trade Commission. (1984). *Statement on false and deceptive advertising practices.* Government Printing Office: Washington, DC.

Fletcher, J. (1966). *Situation ethics: The new morality.* Philadelphia: The Westminster Press.

Florida Statute, Ann 458.331 (1) (o) (West 1981).

General Accounting Office. (December, 1988). Physician incentive payments by prepaid health plans cause lower quality of care. Report to the Chairman, Subcommittee on Health, Committee on Ways and Means, United States House of Representatives. Washington, DC: Government Printing Office.

General Assembly of the World Medical Association. (1948). *Declaration of Geneva.*

Gray, B.H. (1986). *For profit enterprise in health care.* Washington, DC: National Academy Press.

Gregory, J. (1817). *Lectures on the duties and qualifications of a physician.* Philadelphia: M. Varney & Son.

Gunn, A.S., & Vesilind, P.A. (1990). Why can't you ethicists tell me the right answers? *Journal of Professional Issues in Engineering, 116*(1), 9–15.

Harford, E. (1991, September-October). *Audiology Today, Bulletin of the American Academy of Audiology, 3*(5), 29–31.

Hauerwas, S. (1986). *Suffering presence: Theological reflections on medicine, the mentally handicapped, and the church.* Notre Dame: Notre Dame University Press.

Hill, D. S. (1990, October). Leadership and professional ethics. In *Reflections on ethics: A compilation of articles inspired by the May 1990 ASHA ethics colloquim* (pp. 7–14). Rockville, Maryland: American Speech-Language-Hearing Association.

Hill, I. (1980). *Common sense and everyday ethics.* American Viewpoint, Inc., The Ethics Resource Center, Washington, DC: The Ethics Resource Center.

Hillman, A. (1987). Financial Incentives for Physicians in HMOs: Is There a Conflict of Interest? *New England Jornal of Medicine, 317*(27), 1743–1748.

Hillman, A. (1989). How do financial incentives affect physicians' clinical decisions and the financial performance of health maintenance organizations? *New England Journal of Medicine, 321*(32), 86–92.

Hoppin, M. E. (1987). A university perspective on pharmaceutical and industry support of research. *American Journal of Clinical Nutrition, 46,* 226–228.

Illinois Stat. Ann., Ch. 111, 4433 (18) (Smith-Hurd), 1986.

InterStudy: A mid-year report on HMO growth. (June 1986). Excelsior, MN: InterStudy, Inc.

Issues and Facts. (January, 1992). *Audecibel, XLV,* No. 1.

Kenny, A. (1978). *The Aristotelian ethics.* Clarendon, England: Oxford Press.

King, L. (1982). The old code of medical ethics and some problems it had to face. *Journal of the American Medical Association, 248,* 2329–2333.

Konold, D. (1978). *Codes of medical ethics—history.* New York: Free Press.

Kreuzer v. American Academy of Periodontology, 735 F. 2d, 1479, 1488-89, (D.C. Cir. 1984).

Leary, W.E. (1989, June 12). Business and scholarship: A new ethical quandry. *The New York Times,* p. 12.

Levy, N.I., & Mishkin, D.B. (1990). In whose best interest is it anyway?. In *Reflections on ethics: A compilation of articles inspired by the May ASHA ethics colloquim.* Rockville MD: ASHA.

Luft, H. (1978). How do health maintenance organizations achieve their 'savings'? Rhetoric and evidence. *New England Journal of Medicine, 298,* 1336–1343.

May, W.F. (1975, December). Code, covenant, contract or philanthropy? *Hastings Center: Report 5,* 29–38.

McChesney, F. S. (1985). The law and economics of professional advertising. In *Advertising by Health Care Professionals in the 80s.* Washington, DC: Federal Trade Commission.

McCuen, R.H. (1983). Engineering research: Potential for fraud. *Journal for Professional Issues in Engineering, 109*(3), 185–194.

Michigan, Opinion of the Attorney General. (June 8, 1979). No. 5498.

Missouri, Opinion of the Attorney General. (July 8, 1982). No. 6.

Nash, L. L. (1988). Ethics without the sermon. In *Biomedical ethics, a resource guide.* Tampa, FL: American Academy of Medical Directors.

Natanson v. Kline, 186 Mich. 393; 350 P.2d 1093 (1979).

O'Rourke, K. (1986). Medical ethics: Common ground for understanding. Saint Louis: Catholic Health Association.

Palazzo v. Teasdale et al., No. 11596, (Michigan Ct. App. 1989).

Palca, J. (1989). NIH grapples with conflict of interest. *Science, 242,* 23.

Pellegrino, E.D., & Thomasma D.C. (1988). *For the good of the patient.* New York: Oxford University Press.

Percival, T. (1927). *Percival's medical ethics.* Reprint 1803, Chauncey D. Leake (Ed.). Baltimore: Williams & Wilkins.

Plato. (1957). *The Republic, I,* 342d. New York: Modern Library.

Pope, K., & Bouhoutsos, J. (1986). *Sexual intimacy between therapists and patients.* New York: Praeger.

Pound, R. (1953). *The lawyer from antiquity to modern times.* Reports of the Council on Ethical and Judicial Affairs of the American Medical Association. Chicago: American Medical Association.

President's Commission for the Study of Ethical Problems in Medicine and Biomedical and Behavioral Research. (1983). *Summing Up: Final Report.* Washington, DC: Government Printing Office.

Rahman, Abdul, Amine, C., & Elkadi, A. (1981). Islamic Code of Medical Professional Ethics. Papers Presented to the First International *Conference on Islamic Medicine celebrating the advent of the Fifteenth century Hijri.* Kuwait: Kuwait Ministry of Health.

Reeder, J. P. (1982). Beneficence, supererogation, and role duty. In E. Shelp (Ed.), *Beneficence and health care.* Dordrecht, Germany: Reidel.

Reich, W. (Ed.), (1978). Oath of Initiation. *Encyclopedia of bioethics, 4,* 1732–1733. New York: The Free Press.

Resnick, D.M. (1991). An introduction to ethics. *Audiology Today: Bulletin of the American Academy of Audiology, 3*(5), 13.

Rhode Island General Laws 5-37. 1-5(6) (1985).

Roeder, D., & Shimberg, B. (1986). *Occupational licensing: centralizing state licensing functions.* Lexington, KY: The Council of State Governments.

Schwartz, A. E. (1990). Ethics in engineering. In *Reflections on ethics: A compilation of articles inspired by the May 1990 ASHA ethics colloquim.* Rockville, MD: ASHA

Shaw, G.B. (1965). The doctor's dilemma. Baltimore: Penguin. (Especially note the "Preface on Doctors".)

Shulman v. The Washington Hospital Center, 222 F. Supp 59(D.D.C.)*aff'd* 348 F.2d 70 (D.C.Cir.1963).

Siu, A. (1986). Inappropriate use of hospitals in a randomized Trial of health insurance plans. *New England Journal of Medicine, 315,* 1259–1266.

Stromberg, C. (1988). *The psychologist's legal handbook.* Washington, DC: Council for the National Register.

Stromberg, C. (1990). Key legal issues in professional ethics. In *Reflections on ethics: A compilation of articles inspired by the May 1990 ASHA ethics colloquim.* Rockville, MD: ASHA.

Sweede v. Cigna, No. 87-C-SE-71-1-CV (Delaware Super Ct. 1988.

Teti v. United States Healthcare, 1989 W. L. 14327 (E. D. Pennsylvania). Also see: Sweede v. Cigna, No. 87-C-SE-71-1-CV (Delaware Super. Ct. 1988); Bush v. Dake, No. 86-25767 NM (Mich Cir. Ct. 1988).

Texas Statute Ann., art. 4495 (b) 509 (Vernon 1986).

Titus, H., & Keeton, M. (1978). *Ethics for today*. New York: D. Van Nostrand.

Unschuld, P. (1979). *Medical ethics in Imperial China: A study in historical anthropology*. Berkley, CA: University of California Press.

U.S. Department of Health and Human Services. (1984). Child Abuse and Neglect Prevention and Treatment Program. *Federal Register, 49*, 1622–1654.

U.S. Department of Health and Human Services. (1985). Child Abuse and Neglect Prevention and Treatment Program. *Federal Register, 50*, 14873–14892.

Virginia Code 54-317 (12) (1985).

Veatch, R. (1981). *Medical ethics*. New York: Basic Books.

Vollmer, H., & Mills, D. (Eds.) (1966). *Professionalization*. Englewood Cliffs, NJ: Prentice- Hall.

Waggoner, K. M. (1990). Professional ethics, A methodology for decision-making: Expert systems in the classroom. In *Reflections on ethics: A compilation of articles inspired by the May 1990 ASHA ethics colloquim*. Rockville, MD: ASHA.

Wallace, J. D. (1978). *Virtues and vices*. Ithaca, NY: Cornell University Press.

Wasteful use of Medicare funds. (1990, November 19). *Washington Post*, p. 8.

Webster's new world dictionary: Second edition. (1984). New York: Prentice Hall.

Weiss, P. (1990, December 14). Pharmaceuticals give in. *Washington Post*, p. 11.

Withrow v. Larkin, 421 U.S.35 (1975).

Wolff v. McDonnell, 418 U.S. 539 (1974).

World Medical Association. (1956). Declaration of Geneva. *World Medical Journal,3*(Suppl. 12).

Wright, R. A. (1987). *Human values in health care: The practice of ethics*. New York: McGraw-Hill.

INDEX